Atlas of INFECTIONS OF THE NERVOUS SYSTEM

Atlas of INFECTIONS OF THE NERVOUS SYSTEM

W Edmund Farrar MD
Professor of Medicine and Microbiology
Medical University of South Carolina
Charleston, South Carolina
USA

M WOLFE

Cover pictures
Upper: Perivascular demyelination and mononuclear inflammation in a patient with post-vaccinal encephalomyelitis.
Lower left: India ink preparation of CNS sediment from a patient with cryptococcal meningitis, showing the prominent capsule of the causative organism, *Cryptococcus neoformans.*
Lower right: Post-contrast MRI scan showing a left-sided subdural empyema.

Copyright © 1993 Mosby–Year Book Europe Limited.
Published in 1993 by Wolfe Publishing, an imprint of Mosby–Year Book Europe Limited.

ISBN: 1 56375 615 3

The material in this book is derived from *Infectious Diseases: Text and Color Atlas* by W Edmund Farrar, Martin J Wood, John A Innes and Hugh Tubbs (Gower Medical Publishing, 1991).

Originated in Singapore by ScanTrans.
Printed by Grafos SA Arte Sobre Papel, Spain.
Printed and bound in Spain, 1993.

Cataloguing in Publication data:
CIP catalogue records for this title are available from the British Library and the US Library of Congress.

For full details of all Mosby–Year Book Europe Limited titles, please write to Mosby–Year Book Europe Limited, Lynton House, 7–12 Tavistock Square, London WC1H 9LB, England.

Preface

Infections of the nervous system constitute a remarkably diverse group of conditions, ranging in severity from mild, even asymptomatic, viral aseptic meningitis to potentially devastating illnesses such as brain abscess, herpes simplex encephalitis and rabies. The spectrum of causative microorganisms includes cellular organisms such as bacteria, fungi and protozoa as well as viruses and even simpler 'organisms' of uncertain nature (prions). Because of the vital importance of the nervous system for life and function, and the vulnerability of nervous tissue to injury once its protective barriers have been breached, these infections often have more serious consequences for the human host than those involving other organ systems.

In this realm of medicine as in many others a good illustration may greatly facilitate the understanding of a disease process, or even lead directly to an accurate diagnosis. In this book I have tried to take full advantage of the visual possibilities, and have included clinical photographs, pictures of gross pathology, light and electron micrographs of histopathologic changes and microorganisms, and imaging studies utilizing radiographic and radionuclide techniques. I hope and believe it will be valuable not only to neurologists and neuropathologists, but also to internists, pediatricians and other physicians and clinical workers who encounter these infections in their work.

Acknowledgements

First, I thank my wife Carver, for her constant support, encouragement and help in this endeavor.
This collection of pictures could not have been assembled without the generous collaboration of many friends and colleagues in various parts of the world. I wish to express here my appreciation to all of them; the sources of individual slides are given in the captions.
I am especially grateful to the following individuals: Dr Paul D Garen, who made available extensive neuropathological material and provided much helpful advice; Dr Martin J Wood, a co-author on other occasions, who contributed many valuable illustrations; Drs Pamela Van Tassel and Joel K Curé, who provided most of the radiographic and radionuclide imaging studies, and Drs H Whitwell, G Douglas Hungerford, Thomas F Sellers Jr, and Ms Elena Prevost Smith, who provided valuable pictures not available from other sources.
Finally, at Mosby Europe, Stephen McGrath and Michele Campbell deserve special thanks for their commitment, encouragement and professional skills.

WEF
Charleston, 1993

Contents

Chapter 1

The Central Nervous System:
Anatomy and Infection

The brain and spinal cord are surrounded by three layers of meninges: the pia mater and arachnoid (leptomeninges), and the dura mater (pachymeninges). The pia is applied closely to the brain and cord. It extends into the brain around penetrating vessels and merges with the ependymal lining of the fourth ventricle at the foramina of Luschka and Magendie. Between the pia mater and arachnoid is the subarachnoid space, which contains the cerebrospinal fluid (CSF), in which the brain and spinal cord are suspended. Infection within the subarachnoid space may spread to involve the entire surface of the brain and cord, and may extend through the foramina of Luschka and Magendie to produce *ventriculitis*. The dura and arachnoid are attached at only a few points, so that subdural infection may spread rapidly over an entire cerebral hemisphere to produce a *subdural empyema*. Infection outside the dura is confined by the close attachment of the dura to periosteum and bone, and the result is a localized *epidural abscess*. Below the cervical region of the cord the dura and periosteum are separated by a fat-filled epidural space which offers little resistance to the longitudinal spread of infection; thus both subdural empyema and epidural abscess may extend over many vertebral segments.

Infection in the paranasal sinuses, mastoid or middle ear may spread by direct extension to cause meningitis, abscess, empyema, cranial nerve palsies, optic neuritis or cavernous sinus thrombophlebitis. Cranial nerve palsies, often involving multiple cranial nerves, are especially common in chronic infections of the basilar meninges due to *Mycobacterium tuberculosis* or *Cryptococcus neoformans*.

The blood vessels of the central nervous system (CNS) are the most frequent route by which infection reaches the CNS. Direct involvement of vessel walls, as in septic embolization, or multiplication of organisms in cells of vascular endothelium, as in Rocky Mountain spotted fever, may occur. *Mycotic aneurysm* (bacterial or fungal infection of the vessel wall) may result in infarction or rupture of the vessel wall, with intracranial haemorrhage. The largest amount of blood flow to the brain is through the middle cerebral arteries; thus the likelihood of septic embolization resulting in brain abscess or mycotic aneurysm is greatest in the area supplied by these vessels. Vasculitis of intracranial vessels may occur in hepatitis B virus antigenaemia, meningovascular syphilis, ophthalmic herpes zoster infection or rubella encephalitis. Although most infectious agents reach the CNS by haematogenous spread, neurotropic spread of viruses to the CNS has been demonstrated in herpes simplex virus infections, herpes zoster and rabies.

Infection and inflammation produce loss of capillary integrity, with transudation of intravascular fluid into the brain or cord. Oedema is thus a virtually inevitable consequence of infection in the CNS. Generalized infection within the subarachnoid space may therefore result in an increase in intracranial pressure, but unless severe cerebral oedema, abscess or empyema is present there is little danger of herniation of brain tissue, either spontaneously or following lumbar puncture. Herniation of the temporal lobe through the tentorium cerebelli results in paresis of the third cranial nerve and signs of compression of the corticospinal tract, progressing to coma and loss of brainstem reflexes, finally resulting in respiratory arrest as the medullary respiratory centres are affected. Herniation of the cerebellar tonsils through the foramen magnum may occur, especially in mass lesions of the posterior fossa. Because of its long intracranial course, paresis of the sixth nerve may result from increased intracranial pressure even without direct involvement of the nerve by the inflammatory process.

Chapter 2

Meningitis (I)

Meningitis is defined as inflammation of the meninges, usually but not always due to infection. It may be acute or chronic. Acute meningitis may be purulent (usually bacterial) or aseptic (usually, but not always, viral). Characteristic features of meningitis are stiff neck (Fig. 2.1), and other clinical signs of meningeal irritation and abnormalities of the cerebrospinal fluid (CSF), including pleocytosis (increase in the number of cells), elevation of the protein concentration and (in bacterial, fungal or tuberculous infection) diminished glucose concentration. Fever, headache, mental obtundation and signs of cranial nerve dysfunction may also be present. In purulent meningitis the cells in the CSF are usually predominantly neutrophils. In aseptic meningitis mononuclear cells generally predominate.

ASEPTIC MENINGITIS

Aseptic (non-purulent) meningitis may be caused by a wide variety of agents, but most commonly by viruses. Other infections which may be associated with the acute aseptic meningitis syndrome are leptospirosis, syphilis, tuberculous meningitis and cryptococcal meningitis. With only a few exceptions, which are described below, the clinical picture gives few clues towards an aetiological diagnosis, but the epidemiological setting may be helpful in some cases. Most patients have headache, fever, stiff neck and photophobia.

Distinction between viral and bacterial meningitis depends primarily upon examination of the CSF. In viral meningitis this usually contains from 50–500 leucocytes/mm^3, mainly lymphocytes. Early in the course of the disease there may be a predominance of neutrophils, but within 12–24 hours there is usually a shift to a predominance of lymphocytes. The CSF glucose is normal (above 40 mg/dl) in nearly all cases, but may occasionally be low in infections due to lymphocytic choriomeningitis, herpes simplex or mumps viruses. Protein concentration is usually elevated but is rarely above 200 mg/dl.

Viral Causes

Common viral causes of aseptic meningitis in industrialized countries are echovirus, coxsackievirus, mumps virus, herpes simplex virus and human immunodeficiency virus. In developing countries polioviruses and lymphocytic choriomeningitis virus remain important. In immunocompromised patients meningitis due to cytomegalovirus (CMV; Fig. 2.2) and adenoviruses, often with an associated encephalitis, is sometimes seen.

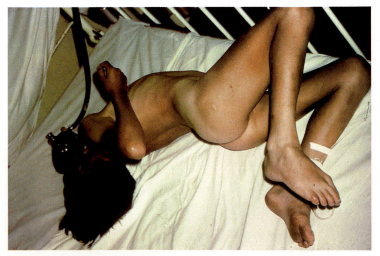

Fig. 2.1 Bacterial meningitis. Severe opisthotonos, due to spasm of muscles of neck, back and extremities. Courtesy of Dr MJ Wood.

Enteroviruses

Enteroviruses are small RNA viruses which are distributed throughout the world. Most serotypes of echoviruses and coxsackieviruses are capable of causing aseptic meningitis. The most common serotypes associated with this syndrome have been echoviruses 4, 6, 9, 11, 16 and 30, and coxsackieviruses A7, A9 and B2–B5. In the northern hemisphere most cases occur in late summer and early autumn. Attack rates are highest in children less than one year old, but meningitis due to these agents is also seen in older children and young adults. Pharyngitis and other symptoms of upper respiratory tract infection may be present.

The disease may be biphasic in course, with signs and symptoms of meningitis occurring several days after the patient has apparently recovered from a non-specific viral illness. Specific aetiological diagnosis of enteroviral meningitis depends upon viral isolation, since serological diagnosis is impractical because of the large number of serotypes. Throat washings, stools and CSF should be cultured. If an agent is isolated, its pathogenic role may be confirmed by demonstrating a rising titre of antibodies after infection.

In areas where poliovirus infections are common, these viruses may cause an illness indistinguishable from that produced by echoviruses and coxsackieviruses. Very rarely, echoviruses and coxsackieviruses have caused the Guillain–Barré syndrome, transverse myelitis or a flaccid motor paralysis, which is usually milder than poliomyelitis and is followed by complete recovery. A chronic, progressive meningo-encephalitis may occur in immunocompromised individuals, especially those with X-linked agammaglobulinaemia.

Except for the vaccines against poliomyelitis, there are no specific vaccines or antiviral agents effective against enteroviral infections. A few cases of persistent infection in immunocompromised individuals have responded to administration of immune globulin.

Mumps virus

Mumps virus is a single-stranded RNA virus of the paramyxovirus family. It is worldwide in distribution, occurring primarily in school-age children and adolescents. Although parotitis is the characteristic manifestation of mumps virus infection, involvement of the central nervous system (CNS) is very common;

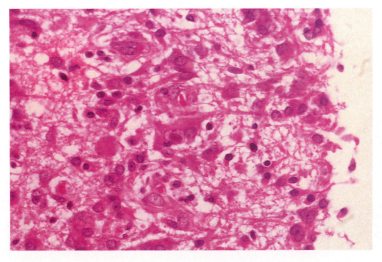

Fig. 2.2 Cytomegalovirus encephalitis. Subependymal cell containing large intranuclear Cowdry type A inclusion of CMV. H&E stain. Courtesy of Dr P Garen.

up to 50% of individuals with mumps but without clinical evidence of meningitis exhibit pleocytosis in the CSF. Clinical meningitis occurs in 1–10% of individuals with mumps parotitis; only about half of patients with mumps meningitis have parotitis. Meningitis usually appears a few days after the onset of the parotitis, but may occur earlier, or as long as two weeks later. As with parotitis, the incidence is higher in men, and most cases are seen in spring and summer. More serious disease of the nervous system, such as encephalitis, deafness, facial palsy, transverse myelitis, Guillain-Barré syndrome or poliomyelitis-like paralysis, is rare. Specific laboratory diagnosis of mumps meningitis is rarely worthwhile but the virus can usually be isolated from saliva, and frequently from CSF, during the first week of illness. Diagnosis may be confirmed by demonstration of a rising titre of antibody in the serum.

Herpes simplex virus

The most serious form of disease of the nervous system caused by herpes simplex viruses is encephalitis (see Chapters 5 and 6), usually due to type 1 virus, but type 2 virus can also cause meningitis. Meningitis is a common complication of primary genital herpes virus infection, especially in women; up to 36% of women and 13% of men have headache, nuchal rigidity and photophobia. CSF pleocytosis is often found in those ill enough to have lumbar puncture. Meningitis also occurs as a component of disseminated infection in newborn infants of women with active genital herpes virus infection. Sacral radiculopathy, with sacral paraesthesias, urinary retention and constipation, or transverse myelopathy, may also occur.

Lymphocytic choriomeningitis virus

Human infection with lymphocytic choriomeningitis virus (LCMV) is associated with exposure to rodents and their urine. Most sporadic cases are attributed to contact with infected mice (*Mus musculus*), and all reported outbreaks have been traced to contact with infected Syrian hamsters. The clinical picture differs from that seen in the usual case of aseptic meningitis. Initially, there is a non-specific febrile illness, sometimes with a maculopapular rash and lymphadenopathy. This subsides, and is followed within a few days by the onset of severe headache, elevated CSF pressure and occasionally papilloedema. Only a minority of patients exhibit signs of meningitis. Rarely orchitis, mild pericarditis or arthritis may occur. The second phase of the illness coincides with the appearance of antibody, and may represent an immunological phenomenon. Diagnosis may be made by demonstrating a rise in

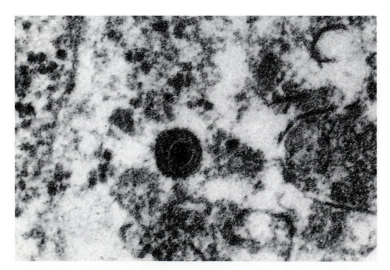

Fig. 2.3 Electron micrograph of an HIV particle with a rounded, central nucleus.

antibody titre or by intracerebral inoculation of mice with blood or spinal fluid followed in one week by the injection of endotoxin, which precipitates illness in infected mice. Except for prevention of contact between humans and rodents by community rodent control programmes, there are no effective preventive measures against LCM infection.

Human immunodeficiency virus

Aseptic meningitis may occur during infection with the human immunodeficiency virus (HIV; Fig. 2.3). It is a component of the acute retroviral syndrome, which occurs around the time of seroconversion in approximately 25% of patients (Figs 2.4 & 2.5). An acute or subacute meningitis, lasting days to months, may also occur later in the course of HIV infection, with or without evidence of immunodeficiency.

Bacterial Causes

Leptospirosis

In leptospirosis, aseptic meningitis is a common manifestation of the second, or immune, stage of the disease. Although leptospires may be found in the CSF during the first non-specific febrile stage of leptospirosis, they disappear during the second week with the appearance of serum antibody. CSF pleocytosis occurs in 80–90% of patients during the second week of illness and half of these exhibit clinical signs of meningitis. A biphasic illness or history of contact with animals may provide clues to the diagnosis; otherwise the meningitis is non-specific in its manifestations. In the USA leptospirosis probably accounts for approximately 10% of cases of aseptic meningitis. The meningitis lasts usually only a few

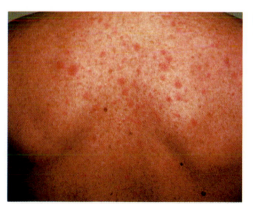

Fig. 2.4 Maculopapular truncal rash occurring during the acute retroviral syndrome. Courtesy of Dr BK Fisher.

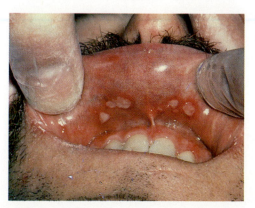

Fig. 2.5 Oral aphthous ulcers occurring during the acute retroviral syndrome. Courtesy of Dr G Griffin.

days (rarely 2–3 weeks) and virtually all anicteric patients recover. Specific diagnosis may be made by demonstration of leptospires in the blood or CSF during the first stage of the illness or in the urine during the second stage, or by retrospective demonstration of a rising titre of antibody. Since the prognosis is uniformly favourable in anicteric cases, antibiotic therapy is probably not indicated, but recent studies show that therapy with penicillins or tetracyclines is beneficial in severe cases.

Syphilis

Aseptic meningitis may occur in syphilis, especially during the secondary stage, and may be the first manifestation of infection with *Treponema pallidum.* Papilloedema, cranial and peripheral neuropathies, mental deterioration and seizures are more frequent in syphilitic than in viral meningitis. Although most cases present during the first year after infection, meningitis may occur months or years later. Recent studies show that up to a third of patients with untreated primary or secondary syphilis have *T. pallidum* organisms in the CSF; both serum and CSF serological studies should be performed whenever syphilis is a possible cause of aseptic meningitis syndrome. Older treatment regimens for neurosyphilis utilizing intramuscular penicillin may be inadequate; currently, aqueous penicillin G, 12–24 million units per day (2–4 million units every 4 hours) given intravenously for 10–14 days, is recommended.

Non-infectious Causes

Non-infectious (or presumed non-infectious) causes of this syndrome include the following: carcinomatous involvement of the meninges; chemical irritation; Mollaret's meningitis; Behçet's syndrome; Vogt–Koyanagi–Harada syndrome; sarcoidosis; lupus erythematosus; and many drugs.

Chapter 3

Meningitis (II)

BACTERIAL MENINGITIS

Bacterial meningitis occurs when pathogenic bacteria reach the cerebrospinal fluid (CSF) via the bloodstream, or following direct entry into the subarachnoid space through trauma or other tissue injury. In order to reach the subarachnoid space via the blood, the microorganisms must colonize the nasopharyngeal mucosal epithelium, invade and survive in the intravascular space, cross the blood–brain barrier and survive and multiply in the CSF. The mucosal epithelium is protected by the presence of secretory IgA, but most clinical isolates of the major meningeal pathogens (*Streptococcus pneumoniae*, *Haemophilus influenzae* and *Neisseria meningitidis*) secrete IgA proteases, which cleave the hinge region of this immunoglobulin. The bacteria adhere to mucosal cells and invade the epithelium by various mechanisms to reach the intravascular space. Once inside the intravascular space the microorganisms must evade humoral defence mechanisms, primarily the alternative complement pathway, which does not require specific antibody for activation. From the blood, bacteria penetrate the blood–brain barrier

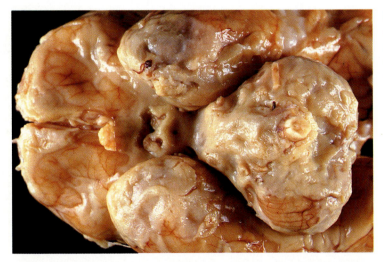

Fig. 3.1 Bacterial meningitis. Gross specimen with copious subarachnoid purulent exudate covering base of brain and enveloping brainstem and cerebellum. Courtesy of Dr P Garen.

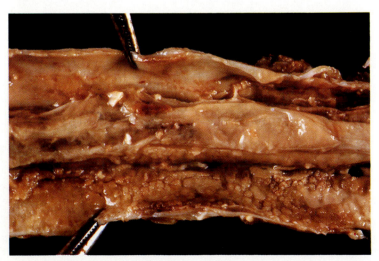

Fig. 3.2 Bacterial meningitis. Spinal cord obscured by thick subarachnoid purulent exudate. Courtesy of Dr P Garen.

formed by capillary endothelium and enter the CSF. Humoral defences in blood, including immunoglobulins and complement components, are lacking from CSF, and the subarachnoid space provides few surfaces against which polymorphonuclear (PMN) leucocytes can trap bacteria in order to ingest them.

Once the microorganisms are inside the subarachnoid space, two bacterial components are chiefly responsible for the stimulation of the inflammatory response, i.e. the breakdown of the blood–brain barrier and passage of leucocytes into the CSF. These are the cell wall (inner membrane) and lipopolysaccharide (outer membrane in Gram-negative bacteria). Mediators of the inflammatory response include tumour necrosis factor (TNF), interleukin-1 (IL-1) and IL-6. These cytokines, made by host cells, are the direct cause of the disease process, meningitis.

Intracranial pressure may increase because of the entry of fluid and inflammatory cells into the subarachnoid space and by the development of oedema of the brain. The latter may cause herniation of brain tissue through the tentorium cerebelli or the foramen magnum. Production of oxygen intermediates in the walls of small blood vessels may result in the loss of normal autoregulation of cerebral blood flow; damage to brain tissue can occur from either hyperperfusion or hypoperfusion.

Although bactericidal antibiotics which can readily enter brain tissue and CSF may rapidly kill the invading microorganisms, death or permanent neurological damage may result from the inflammatory reaction itself. Both experimental and clinical studies support the conclusion that concomitant adjunctive therapy with corticosteroids may improve the clinical response to antibiotics, at least in children. Other anti-inflammatory agents which have actions different from those of corticosteroids, such as pentoxifylline (a phosphodiesterase inhibitor), and monoclonal antibodies directed against the individual components of the inflammatory response, may also prove to be useful as adjunctive agents in the treatment of bacterial meningitis.

Bacteria causing meningitis usually reach the meninges via the blood stream. The three most common bacterial causes of meningitis outside the neonatal period (*S. pneumoniae*, *N. meningitidis* and *H. influenzae*) all inhabit the mucosal surface of the nasopharynx; meningitis is frequently associated with bacteraemia originating at this site. Pneumococcal meningitis also often occurs with pneumococcal pneumonia, and by direct extension from infection of the paranasal sinuses or via skull fracture with communication between the nasopharynx and the subarachnoid space. Multiplication of bacteria in the subarachnoid space causes intense vascular congestion and the formation of a purulent exudate over the surface of the brain (Fig. 3.1) and spinal cord (Fig. 3.2), especially in the sulci (Fig. 3.3) and at the base of the brain (Fig 3.4).

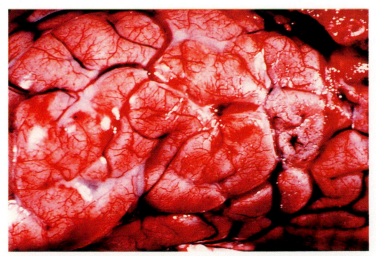

Fig. 3.3 Bacterial meningitis. Gross specimen of fresh brain, revealing intense acute congestion of meningeal blood vessels and purulent exudate in sulci.

Microscopically, the exudate is seen to consist of acute inflammatory cells (Fig. 3.5), in this case confined to the subarachnoid space, contained by the arachnoid membrane on the outermost surface and the pia mater on the innermost surface close to the cerebral cortex. Vascular involvement may be extensive. Thin-walled veins may be infiltrated by PMN leucocytes, and fibrin strands may be seen emanating from the walls (Fig. 3.6). Arteries may show infiltration of PMN leucocytes into the wall with accumulation of these cells beneath the endothelial lining (Fig. 3.7), sometimes narrowing or even occluding the lumen (endarteritis obliterans). In some cases petechial haemorrhages may occur, especially in the cerebral cortex (Figs 3.8 & 3.9). Gram-negative bacillary meningitis, most commonly seen

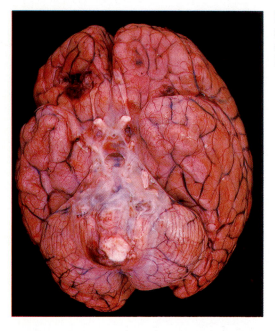

Fig. 3.4 Pneumococcal meningitis. Gross specimen of brain showing accumulation of thick exudate at the base, in a patient who developed meningitis following a basal skull fracture. Courtesy of Dr H Okazaki and Dr BW Scheithauer.

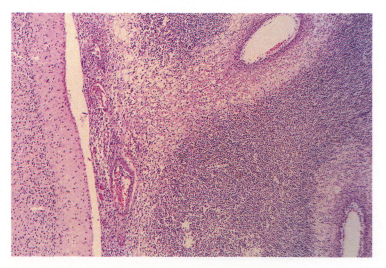

Fig. 3.5 Bacterial meningitis. Intense subarachnoid acute inflammatory exudate in bacterial meningitis. Note lack of involvement of underlying brain. H&E stain. Courtesy of Dr P Garen.

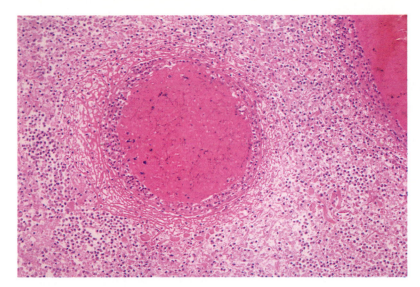

Fig. 3.6 Bacterial meningitis. Thin-walled venous channels infiltrated by polymorphonuclear leucocytes and fibrin strands emanating from the walls. H&E stain. Courtesy of Dr H Okazaki and Dr BW Scheithauer.

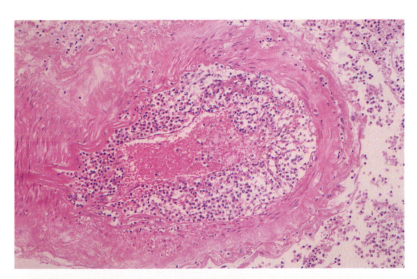

Fig. 3.7 Bacterial meningitis. Section showing artery with infiltration of inflammatory cells beneath the endothelial lining narrowing the lumen (endarteritis obliterans). H&E stain. Courtesy of Dr H Okazaki and Dr BW Scheithauer.

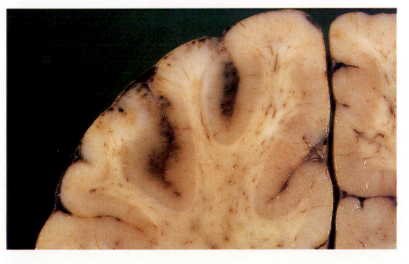

Fig. 3.8 Bacterial meningitis. Gross specimen showing haemorrhages from small blood vessels. Courtesy of Dr H Okazaki and Dr BW Scheithauer.

in neonates and in the elderly, may be associated with necrotizing vasculitis (Fig. 3.10). Ventriculitis, due to multiplication of bacteria in the ventricular system, is present (Fig. 3.11).

Bacterial meningitis often progresses rapidly and patients usually seek medical attention less than 24 hours after the onset of symptoms. Most patients have headache, signs of meningeal irritation, and altered consciousness with or without focal neurological signs. CSF usually exhibits an increased cell count (>1000/mm³), with predominance of PMN leucocytes, an increased protein concentration (>150 mg/dl) and decreased glucose concentration (<40 mg/dl). (If either papilloedema or focal neurological deficits are found on physical examination, lumbar puncture should be delayed until CT or MRI examination is performed, in order to exclude the presence of a mass lesion, with increased risk of herniation of the brain.) Gram stain of the sediment of centrifuged CSF reveals organisms in nearly 90% of patients in whom bacterial cultures are positive (Figs 3.12 & 3.13). Prior antibiotic therapy reduces the yield of both culture and Gram-stain examination, but results of cell count, protein and glucose mea-

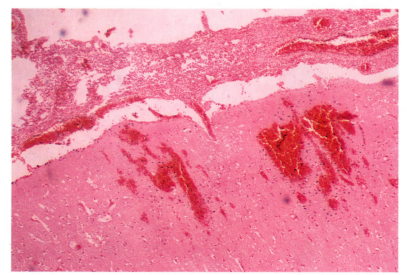

Fig. 3.9 Bacterial meningitis. Microscopic section showing petechial haemorrhages around small blood vessels. H&E stain. Courtesy of Dr H Okazaki and Dr BW Scheithauer.

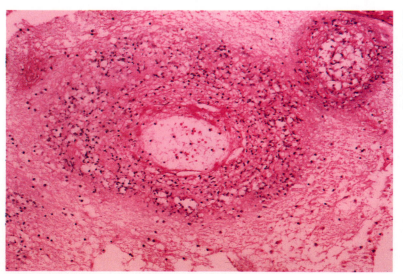

Fig. 3.10 Bacterial meningitis. Microscopic section showing necrotizing vasculitis in infection caused by Gram-negative bacilli. H&E stain. Courtesy of Dr H Okazaki and Dr BW Scheithauer.

surement are usually unaltered, unless the patient has received treatment for several days before examination of the CSF. In previously treated patients, counterimmunoelectrophoresis and latex agglutination tests may provide a specific aetiological diagnosis even though the culture is negative.

Neisseria meningitidis

Meningococcal meningitis occurs most commonly in children and young adults. The infection is worldwide in distribution; most cases occur in winter and spring. *Neisseria meningitidis* is a bean shaped,

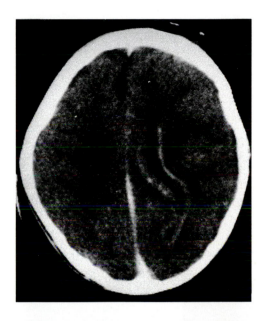

Fig. 3.11 Bacterial meningitis. CT scan showing enhancement of the ependyma of the right lateral ventricle as seen in the ventriculitis complicating bacterial meningitis. Courtesy of Dr GD Hungerford.

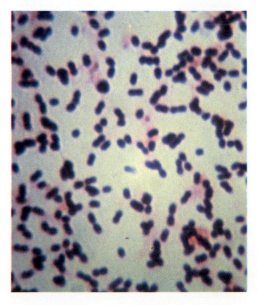

Fig. 3.12 Pneumococcal meningitis. Large numbers of Gram-positive diplococci in cerebrospinal fluid with only a few fragments of degenerating polymorphonuclear leucocytes. Gram's stain. Courtesy of Dr TF Sellers, Jr.

oxidase-positive (Fig. 3.14), Gram-negative diplococcus which inhabits the mucosal surface of the human nasopharynx and is transmitted by respiratory secretions. Of the nine serogroups of *N. meningitidis*, groups A, B, C and Y are responsible for most infections. Asymptomatic nasopharyngeal carriage of *N. meningitidis* is much more common than clinical disease. Its incidence varies greatly among different communities and at different times, and is not closely correlated with the incidence of meningitis. The duration of nasopharyngeal carriage ranges from a few weeks to more than two years and, after weeks or months, often results in the development of protective immunity against clinical illness.

Concomitant viral or mycoplasmal respiratory infection may increase the likelihood of bacteraemic spread from the nasopharynx to the meninges. Except in young infants and the very old, meningococcal meningitis usually presents with headache, confusion and stiff neck. Focal neurological signs and seizures are less common in meningococcal meningitis than in meningitis due to *S. pneumoniae* or *H. influenzae*; this correlates with the rarity of focal cerebral involvement found at autopsy in fatal cases of meningococcal infection. Meningitis is often accompanied by an intense bacteraemia, with production of septic shock, petechiae and purpuric lesions on the skin (Fig. 3.15), peripheral gangrene

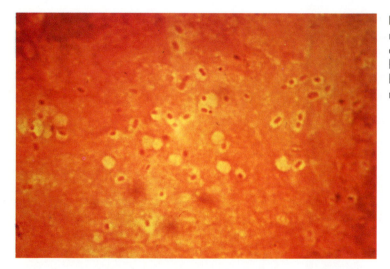

Fig. 3.13 *Klebsiella pneumoniae* meningitis. Gram stain of cerebrospinal fluid showing many heavily encapsulated Gram-negative bacilli and much proteinaceous material. Courtesy of Dr VE Del Bene.

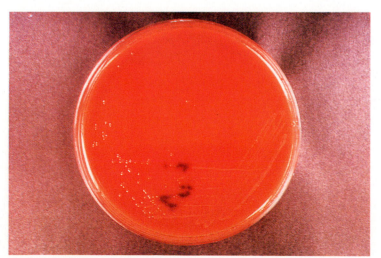

Fig. 3.14 *Neisseria meningitidis.* Oxidase test on chocolate agar. All members of this genus give a positive oxidase test. The reagent (tetramethyl-p-phenylenediamine hydrochloride) is spread over the plate. The colonies of *Neisseria* turn purple.

(Fig. 3.16), and widespread vascular lesions of internal organs including haemorrhagic infarction of the adrenal glands, renal cortical necrosis and disseminated intravascular coagulation.

Strains of *N. meningitidis* are susceptible to many antibiotics (most respond to penicillin G and third-generation cephalosporins), but overwhelming infection may result in death in spite of appropriate therapy. Rare strains of relatively penicillin-insensitive *N. meningitidis* have been found. The treatment of choice is large intravenous doses of penicillin G or a third-generation cephalosporin. Effective antibiotic therapy has reduced the case-fatality rate from more than 70% to less than 10%.

Nasopharyngeal carriage rates of *N. meningitidis* are greatly increased in household contacts of patients and in certain closed populations during epidemics, and household contacts have been shown to have a greatly increased attack rate of meningitis. Elimination of meningococci from most nasopharyngeal carriers can be achieved by administration of rifampin (600 mg twice daily for two days). A quadrivalent vaccine containing polysaccharides of groups A, C, Y and W-135 is now available for immunoprophylaxis in epidemic situations. Children under the age of two years respond poorly to meningococcal vaccines, and there is no effective vaccine against group B strains.

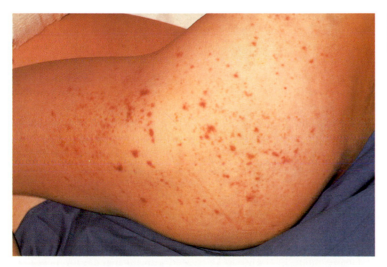

Fig. 3.15 Acute meningococcaemia. Purpuric lesions of variable size on the buttocks and thighs.

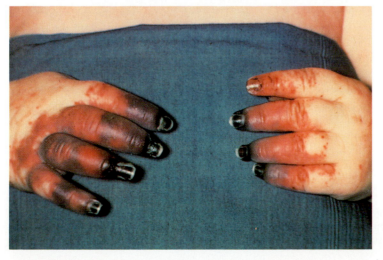

Fig. 3.16 Gangrene of the extremities following a near-fatal illness with hypotension.

Haemophilus influenzae

Haemophilus influenzae is a small, Gram-negative coccobacillus which inhabits the upper respiratory tract of humans. Most cases of meningitis are due to type b strains and occur in children under the age of two years; the disease is rare over the age of six years, but occasional cases are seen in elderly individuals. In spite of this age limitation, in the USA as in many other countries the attack rate is greater than that for any other type of bacterial meningitis. Onset of meningitis is often preceded by evidence of an upper respiratory infection. The clinical picture resembles that of bacterial meningitis of any cause. Because it is a disease of young children, subdural effusion is a common complication (Fig. 3.17). Serious neurological sequelae persist in about half of the patients who recover. Approximately 20% of strains of *H. influenzae* produce a plasmid-mediated β-lactamase and are resistant to ampicillin. Standard therapy consists of chloramphenicol plus ampicillin, given intravenously in large doses. If the strain is found to be susceptible to ampicillin, treatment can be continued with ampicillin alone. Recent studies show that third-generation cephalosporins such as ceftriaxone and cefotaxime are effective in the treatment of meningitis due to this organism. Administration of corticosteroids reduces the incidence of hearing loss in children with meningitis due to *H. influenzae*. Conjugate vaccines, consisting of type B polysaccharide complexed with either nontoxic diphtheria toxoid or *N. meningitidis* outer membrane proteins, are immunogenic in children aged two months or older and are recommended for routine use. For individuals with congenital or acquired hypogammaglobulinaemia, passive immunization may be achieved by intravenous administration of gamma globulin every three weeks. Chemoprophylaxis with rifampin is recommended for all household contacts (children and adults), where the household contains children (other than the index case) less than four years old; such chemoprophylaxis is also recommended in nurseries and day-care centres. A patient returning from hospital to a household in which there are other young children should also receive rifampin in order to eradicate the nasopharyngeal carrier state.

Streptococcus pneumoniae

Streptococcus (formerly *Diplococcus*) *pneumoniae* is a Gram-positive coccus which typically appears as a lancet-shaped encapsulated diplococcus in clinical material (see Fig. 3.12). Pneumonia is the most common type of serious pneumococcal infection, but *S. pneumoniae* is also the most common cause of bacterial meningitis in adults over the age of 30. The disease is especially prevalent in the very young and the very old, and in individuals who have predisposing factors such as sickle cell disease, asplenia, alcoholism, multiple myeloma, chronic lymphocytic leukaemia, agammaglobulinaemia and concomitant endocarditis, pneumonia, sinusitis or otitis media due to *S. pneumoniae*. The organism may reach the meninges via the blood stream from a pneumonic focus or endocarditis. It can also arrive by direct extension from infection in the paranasal sinuses or mastoid, or through a skull fracture with communication between the nasopharynx and the subarachnoid space. The clinical picture and CSF profile are similar to those observed in other forms of bacterial meningitis. The incidence of coma and focal neurological deficits is relatively high in meningitis due to *S. pneumoniae*, and the mortality rate is especially high in neonates and in adults over the age of 40. Depending upon the geographic area, a variable proportion of strains of *S. pneumoniae* is relatively resistant to penicillin G (MIC >0.1μg/ml), so all clinically significant isolates should be tested for susceptibility to penicillin with oxacillin disks. Less commonly, strains resistant to more than 2μg/ml are encountered. Such highly resistant strains were found initially in South Africa, but more recently they have been isolated in many other countries. Infections due to penicillin-susceptible strains may be treated with large doses of penicillin G given intravenously, but those due to more resistant strains should be treated with third-generation cephalosporins such as cefotaxime or ceftriaxone. Patients allergic to penicillin may be given chloramphenicol. A 23-valent vaccine containing capsular polysaccharides of the pneumococcal types most frequently involved in serious systemic infections is available, and is recommended for healthy adults over the age of 65 and several categories of adults and children at high risk for pneumococcal disease.

Other Gram-negative Bacilli

Meningitis due to Gram-negative bacilli (excluding neonatal meningitis and infections caused by *H. influenzae*) has increased in frequency in recent years. Most cases occur in association with neurosurgical procedures, head trauma or bacteraemia originating from a distant focus. The organisms most frequently involved are *Klebsiella pneumoniae* (see Fig. 3.13), *Escherichia coli* and *Pseudomonas aeruginosa*. The clinical picture resembles that seen in other forms of bacterial meningitis, except as it may be modified by the underlying condition of the patient. Introduction of the third-generation cephalosporins has greatly improved the therapy of Gram-negative bacillary meningitis. One of these agents should be given intravenously in maximum dosage, probably in combination with an aminoglycoside. If *P. aeruginosa* is suspected, ceftazidime should be selected. If for any reason a third-generation cephalosporin cannot be used, the regimen should include an aminoglycoside given by the intraventricular route via an Ommaya reservoir as well as intravenously. Bacteriological and clinical response may be slow, and treatment should be continued for at least ten days after the cultures of the CSF become negative. Acute or chronic meningoencephalitis occurs rarely in patients with brucellosis.

Listeria monocytogenes

Listeria monocytogenes usually causes meningitis in neonates or in immunocompromised older children and adults. In neonates the source of the organism is the genital tract of the mother. The Gram-positive rods found on culture of the CSF resemble diphtheroids (Fig. 3.18), and may well be discarded as contaminants from the skin unless the clinician communicates the suspicion of meningitis to the laboratory personnel. A characteristic tumbling motility and β-haemolysis on blood agar aid in the correct identification of *L. monocytogenes*. Both ampicillin plus aminoglycoside, given in large doses intravenously, and trimethoprim–sulphamethoxazole have been used successfully in the treatment of listeria meningitis.

Bacterial Meningitis in Neonates

Bacterial meningitis in the neonatal period differs in several respects from the disease seen in older children and adults. Signs and symptoms pointing specifically to meningeal infection may be lacking. A small number of polymorphonuclear leucocytes and an 'elevated' protein concentration may be present normally in the CSF of neonates and the glucose concentration may not be definitely abnormal even in the presence of infection. The most common

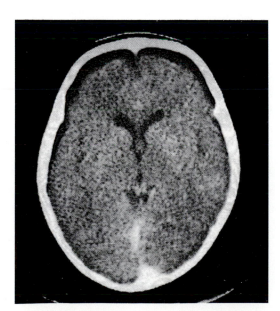

Fig. 3.17 Bacterial meningitis. CT scan showing subdural effusion in frontal region in a patient with meningitis due to *Haemophilus influenzae*. Courtesy of Dr GD Hungerford.

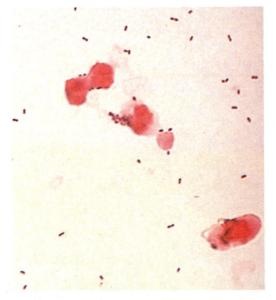

Fig. 3.18 Listeria meningitis. *Listeria monocytogenes* in CSF. Gram's stain. Courtesy of Dr K Nye.

infecting organisms are *E. coli*, group B streptococci, enterococci and *L. monocytogenes*, all components of the vaginal and perineal flora of the mother. Group B streptococci (*Streptococcus agalactiae*) cause two distinct types of meningitis in neonates. Early-onset meningitis occurs during the first five days after birth, often within the first 24 hours, and is frequently associated with obstetric complications and/or prematurity. These infants exhibit signs of respiratory distress, lethargy, poor feeding, fever and

jaundice, but not meningitis; the diagnosis can be made only by examination of the CSF. Late-onset meningitis appears between seven days and three months after birth, at a mean age of approximately three weeks. Serotype III accounts for 95% of late-onset infections. This type of infection usually occurs in term infants and is rarely associated with maternal obstetric complications. These organisms are uniformly susceptible to penicillin G and this is the drug of choice when the aetiological diagnosis has

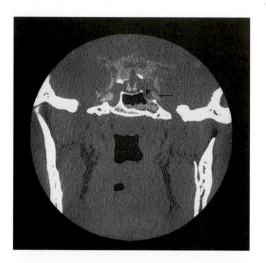

Fig. 3.19 CSF rhinorrhoea. Coronal image from a CT cisternogram in a patient with atrumatic left sided CSF rhinorrhoea. Note the dehiscent left lateral wall of the sphenoid sinus (arrowed). Opacified CSF enters the sphenoid sinus from the CSF space in meckel's cave (arrowed). Courtesy of Dr P Van Tassel.

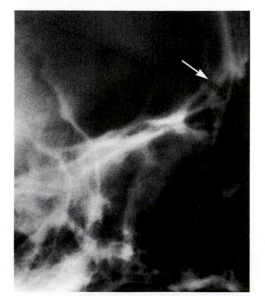

Fig. 3.20 Recurrent bacterial meningitis. Lateral skull film showing fracture through the cribriform plate (arrow). Courtesy of Dr GD Hungerford.

been established. Most authorities recommend initial therapy with ampicillin plus an aminoglycoside for suspected neonatal group B streptococcal infection, because of the synergistic effect of this combination on these organisms.

Other Sources of Bacterial Meningitis

Meningitis in patients with ventriculoatrial or ventriculoperitoneal shunts represents another special case. Coagulase-negative staphylococci, *Staphylococcus aureus* and *Propionibacterium acnes*, presumably originating from the patient's skin, are the organisms isolated most frequently, with Gram-negative bacilli and enterococci found occasionally. To cure these infections it is usually necessary to remove the shunt and give appropriate systemic antimicrobial therapy. In a minority of patients, when the antibiotic susceptibilities of the infecting organism and circumstances allow intensive treatment with bactericidal agents given by both intravenous and intraventricular routes, it has been possible to eradicate the infection without removal of the shunt.

Recurrent episodes of bacterial meningitis may be due to communication between the subarachnoid space and the paranasal sinuses (Fig. 3.19), middle ear, nasopharynx or skin. Communication with the paranasal sinuses, middle ear or nasopharynx usually results from fractures of the cribriform plate (Fig. 3.20), paranasal sinuses or petrous portion of the temporal bone. There is often a history of head trauma, sometimes many years previously. In most cases the cause is *S. pneumoniae*, but other bacterial inhabitants of the upper respiratory tract are occasionally found.

An investigation for the presence of CSF rhinorrhoea (Fig. 3.21) or otorrhoea should be carried out, by injecting either contrast material or a radioactive tracer into the lumbar subarachnoid space and testing for its appearance in the nose or ear. Nasal fluid may be tested for glucose content; this is much lower in nasal secretions than in CSF unless meningitis with hypoglycorrhachia is present.

Communication between the subarachnoid space and the skin may be associated with congenital defects such as cranial or lumbosacral midline dermal sinuses (Fig. 3.22), or meningomyelocoele. In these cases the infecting organisms are usually Gram-negative bacilli. Any defects identified should be repaired surgically.

Occasionally, recurrent meningitis results from a persistent parameningeal focus of infection; surgical drainage or removal of the lesion may be necessary. Very rarely, episodes of recurrent meningitis due to intestinal bacteria have been associated with hyperinfection with *Strongyloides stercoralis*.

Tuberculous Meningitis and Tuberculoma

Tuberculous meningitis and tuberculoma may be an isolated event, due to rupture of an asymptomatic cerebral tuberculoma into subarachnoid or ventricular space, or it may be part of the picture of miliary (disseminated) tuberculosis. The latter case prevails

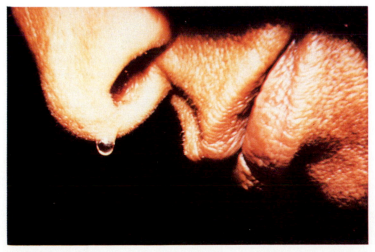

Fig. 3.21 Recurrent bacterial meningitis. Demonstration of cerebrospinal rhinorrhoea. Courtesy of Dr TF Sellers, Jr.

in approximately 75% of patients and evidence of tuberculosis outside the nervous system, most frequently in the lung, can usually be found. When meningitis results from rupture of a solitary subependymal tubercle the diagnosis depends upon findings in the CSF.

The illness may begin acutely but more often the onset is insidious, with gradual development of headache, low-grade fever and signs of meningitis. The chronic meningitis (Figs 3.23, 3.24 & 3.25) is most marked at the base of the brain (Fig. 3.26), and the thick gelatinous exudate often involves cranial

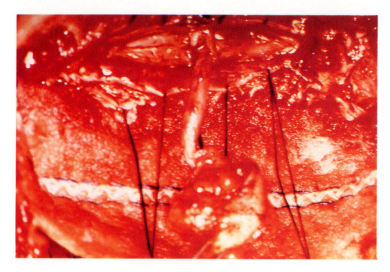

Fig. 3.22 Recurrent bacterial meningitis. Surgical photograph showing a well-defined fistula tract in the sacral region extending from skin to meninges. Courtesy of Dr P Perot.

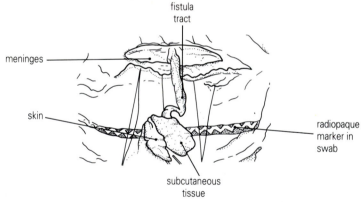

Fig. 3.23 Tuberculous meningitis with granulomatous inflammation. A meningeal vessel demonstrates partial occlusion and organization. Adjacent acute necrosis is apparent. H&E stain. Courtesy of Dr P Garen.

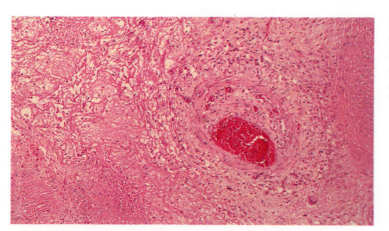

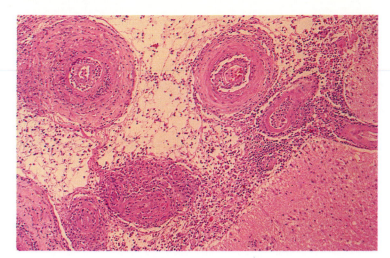

Fig. 3.24 Tuberculous meningitis. Acute tuberculous meningitis with marked involvement of vessel walls and occlusion of smaller vessels. This vascular involvement can result in infarction. H&E stain. Courtesy of Dr P Garen.

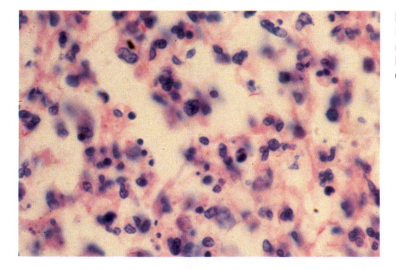

Fig. 3.25 Tuberculous meningitis. Inflammatory exudate containing multiple acid-fast rod-shaped bacilli. Kinyoun–carbolfuchsin stain. Courtesy of Dr P Garen.

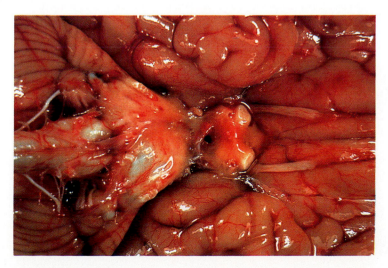

Fig. 3.26 Tuberculous meningitis. Autopsy specimen of a brain showing the thickened gelatinous basal meninges, especially thick in the region of the optic chiasma and over the pons.

nerves (Fig. 3.27) with the production of cranial nerve palsies (Fig. 3.28). As the disease progresses the level of consciousness may be diminished and focal neurological deficits may appear. CSF examination typically reveals pleocytosis with 100–500 cells/mm^3, with predominance of lymphocytes, elevated protein (100–500 mg/ml), and glucose concentration which may be normal or diminished.

Acid-fast bacilli are seen in stained smears of centrifuged CSF in less than a third of patients; the yield may be increased by repeated examinations and by staining the pellicle which forms in the CSF on standing in a test tube. CT scanning or magnetic resonance imaging may reveal the chronic basilar meningitis and tuberculomas within the brain (Fig. 3.29). Tuberculous meningitis may be treated with

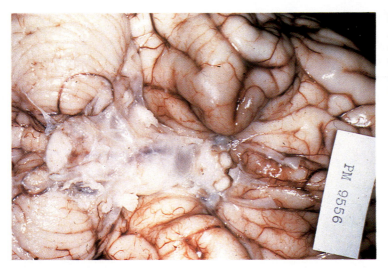

Fig. 3.27 Tuberculous meningitis. Autopsy specimen of the brain of a child showing a sheet of white exudate which encompasses and obscures the basal cranial nerves. Courtesy of Dr JD Balentine.

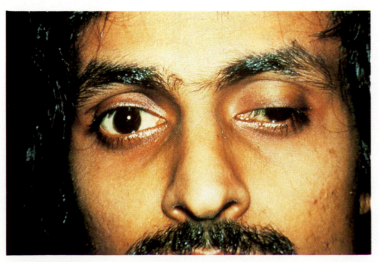

Fig. 3.28 Tuberculous meningitis. Cranial nerve palsies are fairly common. This patient's progress was generally satisfactory but he developed left III paralysis, shown here by ptosis and lateral deviation of the left eye caused by unopposed action of the lateral rectus.

drug regimens effective in the treatment of pulmonary tuberculosis, such as isoniazid plus rifampin for six months, with pyrazinamide given during the first two months. If the level of consciousness is diminished or if focal neurological deficits are present, the addition of corticosteroids for the first few weeks of treatment may be beneficial. Since culture of the organism from CSF may require several weeks, it may be necessary to begin treatment empirically. Clinical improvement after one or two weeks of therapy suggests that the meningitis is indeed due to *Mycobacterium tuberculosis*.

In the absence of meningitis, tuberculomas usually present as space-occupying lesions (Figs 3.30, 3.31, 3.32 & 3.33), often with the onset of seizures. CT scanning usually shows multiple avascular mass

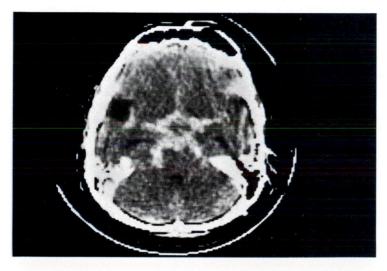

Fig. 3.29 Tuberculous meningitis: CT scan. The vessels of the circle of Willis are thickened and irregular due to contrast enhancement in the inflammatory tissue of the adjacent subarachnoid space. Courtesy of Dr J Ambrose.

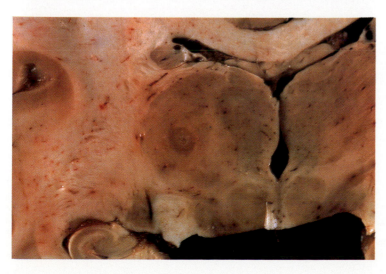

Fig. 3.30 Tuberculoma. Single tuberculous lesion with cavitating necrotic centre present in the thalamus. Courtesy of Dr P Garen.

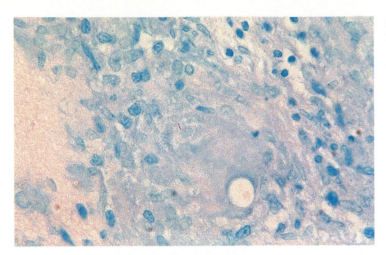

Fig. 3.31 Tuberculoma. Acid-fast bacillus in a granulomatous lesion. Kinyoun–carbolfuchsin stain. Courtesy of Dr H Whitwell.

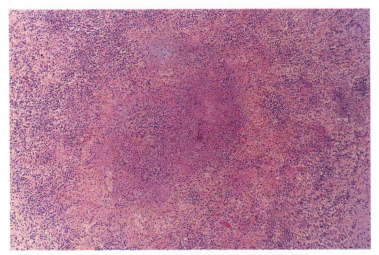

Fig. 3.32 Tuberculoma. Microscopic tuberculoma with central caseation and palisading granuloma. H&E stain. Courtesy of Dr P Garen.

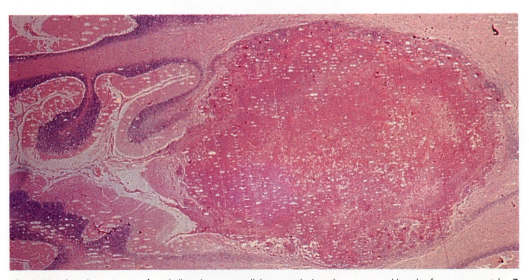

Fig. 3.33 Tuberculoma. Section of cerebellum showing a well-demarcated tuberculoma composed largely of caseous material. × 7. Courtesy of Dr GD Perkin.

lesions surrounded by oedema (Figs 3.34 & 3.35). Isotope scanning may reveal one or more areas of increased uptake (Fig. 3.36). Calcified lesions may be visible on plain films (Fig. 3.37). When the diagnosis is known, therapy with antituberculous drugs should begin; surgery should be avoided if possible, as fewer neurological sequelae result from medical therapy. Concomitant corticosteroid therapy may reduce cerebral oedema and result in an improvement of the symptoms. If the diagnosis is made by biopsy, no further excision should be performed and antituberculous therapy should be instituted.

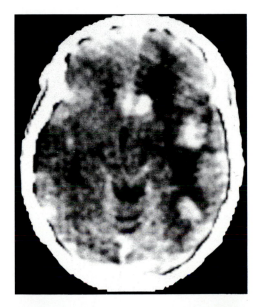

Fig. 3.34 Tuberculoma of the brain. CT scan showing multiple rounded lesions with surrounding oedema. The CT appearance of tuberculoma may be similar to that of pyogenic abscess, a fungal lesion or a meningioma. Courtesy of Dr J Ambrose.

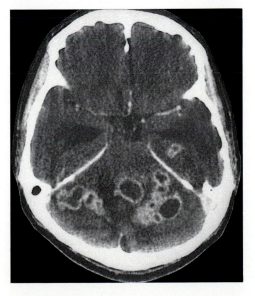

Fig. 3.35 Tuberculoma of the brain. CT scan showing multiple, predominantly ring-enhancing lesions in the cerebellum. Courtesy of Dr GD Perkin.

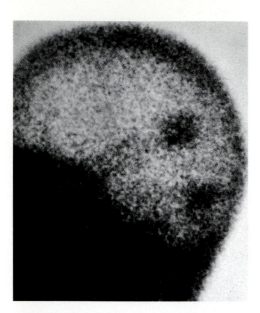

Fig. 3.36 Tuberculoma of the brain. Isotope scan showing two areas of abnormal contrast. The appearance is non-specific but the investigation provides useful information, especially where CT scanning is not available. Courtesy of Dr E Wolinsky.

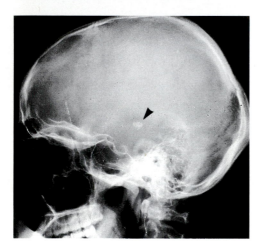

Fig. 3.37 Tuberculoma. Skull radiograph showing a calcified tuberculoma (arrow). Courtesy of Dr GD Perkin.

Chapter 4

Meningitis (III)

FUNGAL MENINGITIS

Cryptococcus neoformans

The yeast-like fungus, *Cryptococcus neoformans,* is by far the most important cause of fungal meningitis. Prior to the era of AIDS about half of patients with cryptococcal meningitis were overtly immunocompromised; Hodgkin's disease, non-Hodgkin's lymphoma and high-dose corticosteroid therapy were the most common underlying conditions. Many apparently immunocompetent individuals exhibit defective cell-mediated immunity to *C. neoformans* following recovery from cryptococcal meningitis;

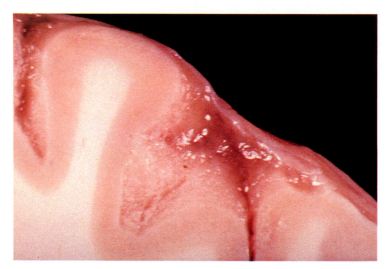

Fig. 4.1 Cryptococcal meningitis. Cross-section of the frontal cortex revealing gelatinous material, which is the capsular material of the organism, in the sulci.

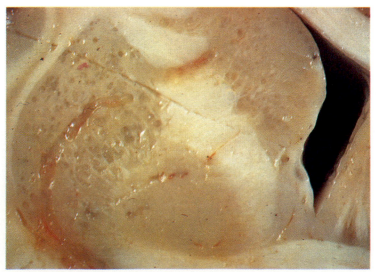

4.2 Cryptococcal meningitis. Gross specimen showing bubble-like lesions in the brain substance. Courtesy of Dr H Okazaki and Dr B Scheithauer.

whether these defects were present prior to the illness or represent a sequela of the infection is not known. Approximately 10% of patients with AIDS develop cryptococcal meningitis; the incidence is even higher in areas where the organism is especially abundant, such as the southeast USA. Pathologically, there is chronic meningitis, often with relatively little inflammatory reaction, as well as scattered cystic lesions comprised of fungal cells embedded in large quantities of the gelatinous polysaccharide capsular material, and distributed deeply within the sulci and in the brain substance (Figs 4.1, 4.2, 4.3, 4.4, 4.5, 4.6 & 4.7).

C. neoformans is worldwide in distribution and appears to be ubiquitous in nature. Humans acquire the organism by inhalation; pulmonary infection,

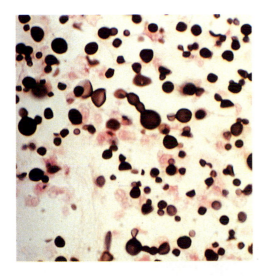

Fig. 4.3 Cryptococcal meningitis. *Cryptococcus neoformans* in exudate within the subarachnoid space. The apparent empty space between the organisms is capsular material. Methenamine silver stain.

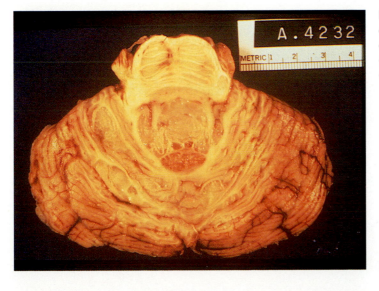

Fig. 4.4 Cryptococcoma. Slice of cerebellum and pons. A large cryptococcoma replaces a major portion of the ventral cerebellar vermis, obliterating the fourth ventricle.

though often inconsequential, is the initial patho-genetic event. The fungus has a special predilection for the meninges, and meningitis may occur as an isolated manifestation or as part of a disseminated infection. The illness often develops gradually with headache, irritability, impairment of memory and judgment, and changes in behaviour. Temperature is sometimes, but not always, elevated, and signs of meningeal inflammation may be minimal or absent. Papilloedema and cranial nerve palsies are relatively

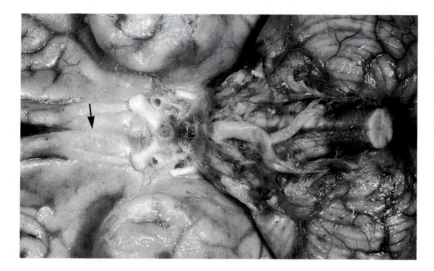

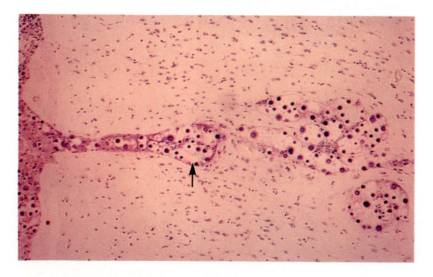

Fig. 4.5 Cryptococcal meningitis. Upper: Opacity of the basal leptomeninges (arrowed). Lower: A section from the same tissue showing cryptococci distending the perivascular space of a cortical blood vessel (arrowed). Nissl stain. × 40. Courtesy of Dr GD Perkin.

common. Except in patients with AIDS, abnormalities are nearly always found in the cerebrospinal fluid (CSF). Typically, there is elevation in the opening pressure, lymphocytic pleocytosis, elevated protein and decreased glucose concentration.

Cryptococci are seen on India ink preparation in approximately 50% of patients. The large polysaccharide capsule of the organism, surrounding the refractile cell wall, gives *Cryptococcus neoformans* a

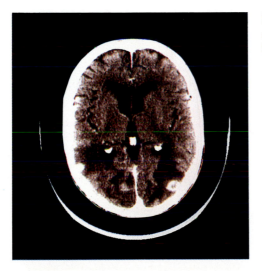

Fig. 4.6 Cryptococcal meningitis. CT scan showing multiple enhancing lesions in the brain, surrounded by oedema. Courtesy of Dr J Curé.

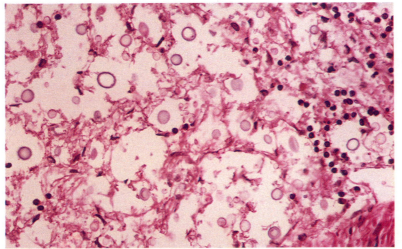

Fig. 4.7 Cryptococcal meningitis. Encapsulated cells of *Cryptococcus neoformans* and mononuclear inflammatory cells in the subarachnoid space. H&E stain. Courtesy of Dr H Okazaki and Dr B Scheithauer.

highly distinctive appearance (Figs 4.8 & 4.9). Cryptococcal polysaccharide antigen is detectable in CSF in 85% of patients, and in serum in approximately 95% of patients.

In patients with AIDS the signs of inflammation in the CSF are drastically diminished: cell count, protein or glucose concentration may be normal in half the patients, and in 20% all three parameters are normal. India ink examination is positive in up to 85% of patients with AIDS, and cryptococcal antigen is found in the CSF in nearly every case. The organism can be cultured from the CSF in virtually all cases, and can often be cultured from other sites, e.g. blood, sputum, urine, faeces or biopsy material.

The standard regimen for treatment of cryptococcal meningitis is the combination of amphotericin B, given intravenously, plus 5-fluorocytosine (flucytosine), administered orally, for at least 6–10 weeks. In patients with AIDS, suppressive treatment with amphotericin B, administered intravenously once weekly for the rest of the patient's life, is relatively effective in preventing recurrence, which is otherwise common. Fluconazole, an antifungal azole which is well absorbed after oral administration, has also been shown to be very effective in preventing recurrence, although it is not very effective in the treatment of cryptococcal meningitis.

Coccidioides immitis

Meningitis due to *Coccidioides immitis* (Fig. 4.10) is virtually limited to individuals living in or travelling through desert areas of the southwestern USA, Mexico and Central and South America, where this

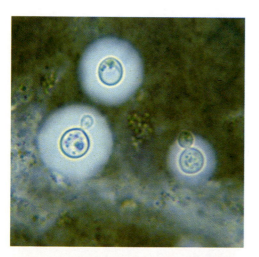

Fig. 4.8 Cryptococcal meningitis. India ink preparation of CSF sediment, demonstrating the prominent capsule of the organism. Note the highly refractile cell wall and internal structure of the yeast. Courtesy of AE Prevost.

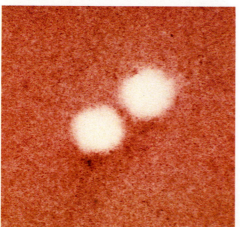

Fig. 4.9 Lymphocytes in CSF sediment. Note that these cells lack the prominent refractile cell wall and internal structure seen in *Cryptococcus neoformans*. India ink preparation. Courtesy of Dr JR Cantey.

fungus is endemic—although a few cases have resulted from exposure to fomites originating in the endemic area. Coccidioidal meningitis may occur as part of a generalized infection or may represent the only extrapulmonary site of disease. The illness may be extremely indolent with headache and minimal signs of meningeal irritation for a long period of time. Examination of the CSF reveals a mononuclear (or rarely eosinophilic) pleocytosis, elevated protein and decreased glucose concentration. Specific aetiological diagnosis is usually made by mycological or serological diagnosis of pulmonary or disseminated coccidioidomycosis, or by finding antibody or the organism in the CSF. Successful treat-

ment of coccidioidal meningitis is very difficult to achieve. Most cures have required combined systemic and either intraventricular or intrathecal administration of amphotericin B for one or two years; some authorities recommend continuation of treatment for the lifetime of the patient. The new azole agents, itraconazole and fluconazole, may simplify the therapy of this disease.

Other Fungal Causes

Rarely, meningitis may be caused by other invasive fungi, such as *Histoplasma capsulatum*, *Blastomyces dermatitidis* (Fig. 4.11) or *Candida albicans* (Figs 4.12 & 4.13), usually as part of a disseminated infection.

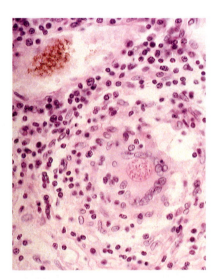

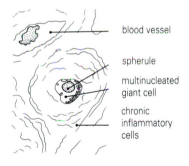

Fig. 4.10 Coccidioidal meningitis. Granulomatous meningitis due to *Coccidioides immitis* showing a multinucleated giant cell containing a spherule of the organism with many endospores. Periodic acid–Schiff stain.

blood vessel

spherule

multinucleated giant cell

chronic inflammatory cells

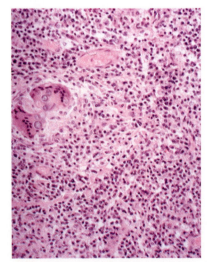

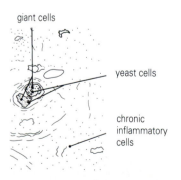

4.11 North American blastomycosis. Granulomatous meningitis with multinucleated giant cells containing *Blastomyces dermatitidis*. H&E stain.

giant cells

yeast cells

chronic inflammatory cells

PARASITIC MENINGITIS

Eosinophilic meningitis may be produced by invasion of the central nervous system (CNS) by larval or adult forms of several species of helminths, including *Angiostrongylus cantonensis* (the rat lung worm), *Gnasthostoma spinigerum* (a human hookworm), *Bayliscaris procyonis* (the raccoon ascarid), *Cysticercus cellulosae* and *Paragonimus westermani*. The diagnosis may be suggested on immunological or clinical grounds, by serological testing or by finding the organism in the CSF. Treatment is the same as that for infection outside the nervous system.

Naegleria fowleri

A rare cause of meningoencephalitis is infection with the free-living amoeba *Naegleria fowleri*. This organism is found worldwide in warm fresh water. Most patients have a history of swimming in fresh water shortly before onset of the illness. After nasal inoculation the amoebae evidently penetrate the submucosal nervous plexus and the cribriform plate to reach the olfactory bulbs and frontal lobes of the brain. There is haemorrhagic necrosis of the olfactory bulbs and contiguous areas of the brain, and eventual development of a diffuse meningoen-

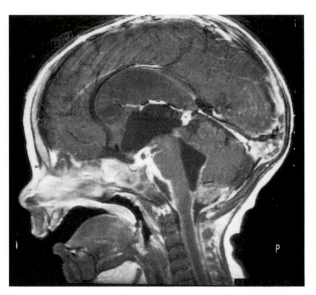

Fig. 4.12 *Candida* meningitis. Sagittal T1-weighted postcontrast MRI in a child with *Candida* meningitis and obstructive hydrocephalus. Note the thick meningeal enhancement in the basal cisterns anterior to the pons, enlarged third and fourth ventricles, and enhancement of surfaces of the cervical spinal cord. Courtesy of Dr P Van Tassel.

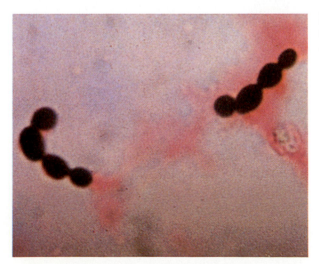

Fig. 4.13 Disseminated candidiasis. Micrograph of CSF sediment showing typical morphology of *Candida albicans*. Gram's stain. Courtesy of AE Prevost.

cephalitis and purulent leptomeningitis. The
trophozoites are found in the olfactory nerves and
around blood vessels in the brain (Fig. 4.14), and an
associated myocarditis may also be seen. The earliest
symptom is often an alteration in taste or smell, followed by the abrupt onset of fever, headache, nausea and vomiting, nuchal rigidity, and alteration in
consciousness. Most patients progress rapidly to
coma and death within a week. The CSF reveals
changes characteristic of purulent meningitis: neu-
trophilic pleocytosis, elevated protein and diminished glucose concentration. Motile trophozoites are
usually found in a wet mount of CSF (Fig. 4.15).

Only two patients are known to have survived primary amoebic meningoencephalitis; both received
high-dose systemic and intrathecal therapy with
amphotericin B; one also received systemic and
intrathecal miconazole and systemic rifampin and
sulphisoxazole.

Acanthamoeba

Focal encephalitis due to one of several *Acanthamoeba* (*Hartmannella*) species is a rare form of
amoebic infection of the nervous system, mainly
seen in immunocompromised patients. In these

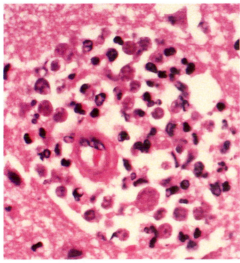

Fig. 4.14 Primary amoebic meningoencephalitis. Upper: Section of
brain showing trophozoites of *Naegleria fowleri* and inflammatory
cells in a Virchow–Robin space from a fatal case in an eight-year-old
child. Lower: Higher power showing the large rounded trophozoites
scattered among inflammatory cells. H&E stains.
Courtesy of Dr S Conradi.

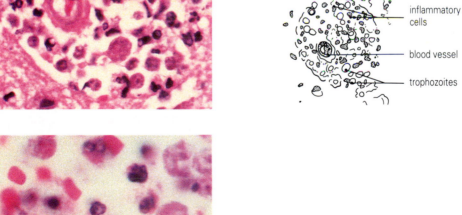

patients, granulomatous skin lesions are present prior to the development of the necrotizing granulomatous lesions in the brain (Fig. 4.16). Brain biopsy is the only method available for making this diagnosis during life. Most cases have been fatal and little is known about therapy. Antimicrobial susceptibility tests have given variable results; pentamidine, ketoconazole, miconazole, and 5-fluorocytosine appear to be more active than amphotericin B against this organism.

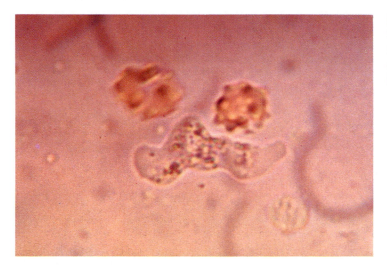

Fig. 4.15 Amoebic meningoencephalitis. Wet mount of CSF sediment showing motile *Naegleria fowleri* from a fatal case in an eight-year-old child. Courtesy of AE Prevost.

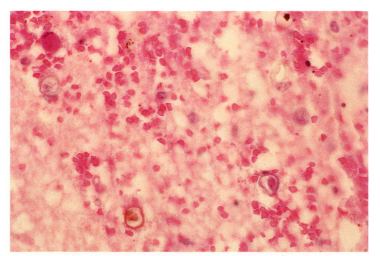

Fig. 4.16 *Acanthamoeba* meningoencephalitis with haemorrhagic necrosis. Organisms with thick irregular capsules and central basophilic nucleus. H&E stain. Courtesy of Dr P Garen.

Chapter 5

Encephalitis (I)

Encephalitis is an inflammation of the brain parenchyma, nearly always a response to invasion by microorganisms, primarily viruses. Frequently, there is concomitant meningitis, so the disease is usually a meningoencephalitis. Depression of consciousness ranging from lethargy to coma, focal neurological deficits and seizures are relatively common.

Clinically, acute viral encephalitis is characterized by the acute onset of fever, headache, stiff neck, depression of consciousness, CSF pleocytosis (predominantly mononuclear) and, frequently, seizures. Focal neurological deficits often develop during the course of the illness.

In fatal cases of viral encephalitis there is usually a prominent perivascular inflammatory reaction composed predominantly of mononuclear cells, although polymorphonuclear leucocytes may also be seen. Evidence of meningitis is also present. Neurons may exhibit degenerative changes, with phagocytosis of neurons by macrophages and microglial cells (neuronophagia) (Fig. 5.1). Inflammatory cells in perivascular areas (and in CSF) are predominantly T-helper cells, with smaller numbers of T-suppressor/cytotoxic cells, B cells and macrophages also present. The distribution of lesions within the nervous system varies among different viral encephalitides. In Japanese B encephalitis there is often extensive infection of brainstem nuclei and structures of the basal ganglia and thalamus; this may explain the frequent occurrence of acute respiratory failure and death in patients with this infection, and the high incidence of dystonic and Parkinsonian sequelae seen in survivors.

RABIES VIRUS

Rabies is a severe viral encephalitis which is nearly always fatal. The virus can infect virtually all mammalian species. Because of geographical isolation, animal control measures and/or quarantine practices, it is absent from many countries including the United Kingdom, Japan, several Scandinavian countries and Australia. Where domestic animal rabies has not been adequately controlled, dogs account for 90% of reported human cases. In areas where rabies in domestic animals is well controlled, such as the USA, Canada and many countries of Western Europe, dogs account for less than 5% of human cases. Cats and certain species of domestic livestock also cause a small proportion of human infections, but a vast reservoir exists in wild mammals. Species which are important in the causation of human rabies in various parts of the world include skunks, raccoons, foxes, wolves, mongooses, jackals and insectivorous and vampire bats. The incidence of human rabies is high in India, the Philippines and many countries in Africa. Most human cases result from bites but well-documented transmission has also occurred via scratches, contamination of mucous membranes with infected saliva, corneal transplantation from a donor with rabies, and inhalation of aerosolized virus in bat caves and in laboratories working with the virus.

The incubation period is usually from a few days up to three months. In a small proportion of cases, the onset of illness occurs between three months and one year. Very rarely, the incubation period is

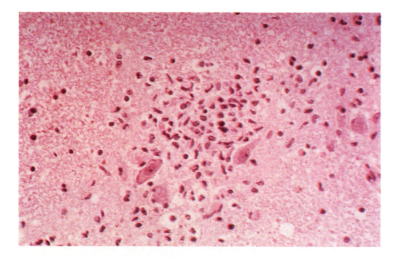

Fig. 5.1 Viral encephalitis. Mononuclear inflammatory cellular response around neurons typical of the so-called 'Babès nodule' associated with viral encephalitis. H&E stain.

from one to five years, or even longer. During most of the incubation period the virus multiplies locally near the site of inoculation, possibly within muscle cells. The virus then spreads via peripheral nerves to the central nervous system (CNS), and by the time symptoms have occurred has travelled outward via efferent pathways to most tissues of the body, including the salivary glands. When symptoms appear, approximately half of the patients have pain or paraesthesia at the inoculation site, but otherwise the manifestations are non-specific and include fever, malaise, fatigue, headache and anorexia. Within a few days neurological manifestations supervene; these may include apprehension, anxiety, agitation, irritability, insomnia, hyperactivity, disorientation, hallucinations, bizarre behaviour, seizures, nuchal rigidity and paralysis. Hyperactivity and delirium are usually intermittent, alternating with periods of orientation and relative calm. Hydrophobia (spasms of the pharynx and larynx provoked by attempts at drinking water, or even by the mere sight of it) or aerophobia (similar effects produced by blowing air on the face of the patient) occur in approximately 50% of cases. A few patients die during this period, but most go on to develop progressive paralysis and eventually coma. To date, only three patients are known to have recovered from rabies, all during the 1970s. Although most cases of human rabies occurring during the last 20 years in the USA and certain other industrialized Western countries have received intensive supportive care, there have been no additional survivors and the disease must still be considered virtually 100%

fatal. Expert intensive care does prolong the period of survival. Potentially fatal complications include respiratory failure, progressive refractory hypoxaemia, seizures and cardiac arrhythmias.

A history of exposure to the rabies virus and a typical clinical picture, especially if hydrophobia and/or aerophobia are present, strongly suggest the diagnosis. Most patients with rabies develop high titres of serum antibody, but individuals who have been immunized with the potent modern human diploid cell vaccines may have titres as high as those seen in clinical rabies. In such patients determination of antibody levels in the CSF may be valuable, since high titres are seen only in clinical disease. The virus has been isolated antemortem from saliva, brain tissue, CSF, urine sediment and tracheal secretions, and postmortem virus isolation has been obtained from many other tissues of the body. Specific immunofluorescent staining of the rabies virus may be accomplished using brain biopsy specimens, corneal impressions or skin biopsy. Histological examination of brain tissue from human cases typically shows perivascular inflammation in grey matter, neuronal degeneration and, in 70–80% of cases, Negri bodies, which are round or oblong eosinophilic cytoplasmic inclusions often containing basophilic spots (Figs 5.2 & 5.3). Immunofluorescent staining of Negri bodies is more sensitive than conventional histological techniques.

Because treatment of rabies is so unsatisfactory, correct post-exposure prophylaxis is extremely important. The physician faced with the decision of whether or not to treat a potential rabies exposure

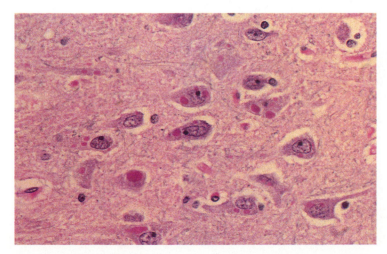

Fig. 5.2 Rabies. Multiple cytoplasmic Negri bodies in hippocampal pyramidal neurons. H&E stain. Courtesy of Dr P Garen.

should obtain specific, current recommendations dealing with this issue and follow them to the letter. Generally speaking, optimal post-exposure prophylaxis includes thorough cleansing of the wound to its deepest extent using a 20% soap solution; active immunization with human diploid cell vaccine, administered intramuscularly in the deltoid region as five 1 ml doses given on days 0, 3, 7, 14 and 28; and a single dose of human rabies immunoglobulin (20 IU/kg), up to half infiltrated around the site of exposure and the remainder given intramuscularly in the gluteal region or anterolateral aspect of the thigh. Individuals at high risk from rabies because of occupation, residence or travel may receive pre-exposure prophylaxis consisting of three 1 ml doses of human diploid cell vaccine given intramuscularly in the deltoid region on days 0, 7 and 21 or 28. Chloroquine phosphate given for malaria chemoprophylaxis may interfere with the development of the antibody response to rabies vaccine.

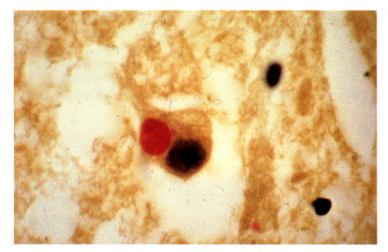

Fig. 5.3 Rabies. Histological section of brain showing a Negri body. H&E stain. Courtesy of Dr MJ Wood.

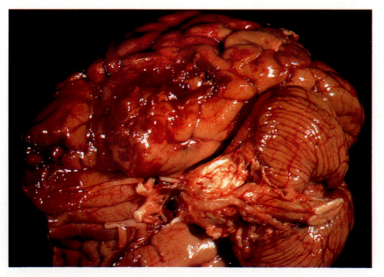

Fig. 5.4 Herpes simplex encephalitis. Gross specimen showing necrosis, haemorrhage and oedema involving the orbital surface of the left frontal lobe and the anterior, medial and lateral surfaces of the left temporal lobe.

HERPES SIMPLEX VIRUS

Herpes simplex encephalitis is a rare complication of herpes simplex infections, but herpes simplex virus (HSV) is one of the most common causes of sporadic acute viral encephalitis in the USA and many other countries. Unlike most other types of infection due to this virus, encephalitis does not seem to be more common in immunocompromised individuals, except perhaps in those with HIV infection. Most cases are due to type 1 virus (HSV-1) but cases occurring during the neonatal period may be due to type 2 virus (HSV-2), acquired from the mother with genital herpes infection. The virus apparently reaches the brain via neural routes during active primary or recurrent infection. Pathologically the infection produces a necrotizing haemorrhagic encephalitis which most commonly involves the temporal lobes (Figs 5.4, 5.5, 5.6 & 5.7). Clinical features often include fever, headache, behavioural disorders, difficulty in speaking and focal seizures. A relatively characteristic feature is olfactory hallucinations. Examination of CSF usually reveals moderate elevation of the protein concentration, normal glucose, and moderate pleocytosis with both mononuclear and polymorphonuclear

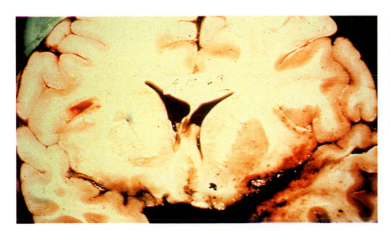

Fig. 5.5 Herpes simplex encephalitis. Coronal section of brain showing haemorrhagic necrosis of the left anterior medial aspect of the left temporal lobe and the orbital surface of the left frontal lobe. This is a characteristic location for the lesion of herpes encephalitis.

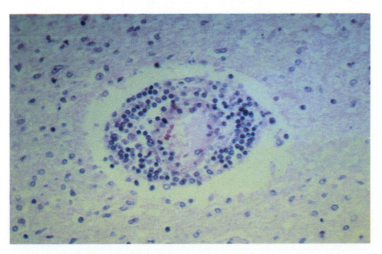

Fig. 5.6 Herpes simplex encephalitis. Perivascular mononuclear inflammatory exudate associated with slight gliosis and inflammation in grey matter of the temporal lobe. H&E stain.

leucocytes. EEG (Fig. 5.8), CT scanning (Fig. 5.9) and MRI (Figs 5.10 & 5.11) often reveal evidence of localized lesions. HSV-1 can rarely be isolated from the CSF, so culture and immunofluorescent staining of brain biopsy specimens (Figs 5.12, 5.13 & 5.14) is the most reliable way to make a specific aetiological diagnosis. Recently, HSV DNA was detected in the CSF in 42 out of 43 proven cases of herpes simplex encephalitis, using a polymerase chain reaction assay. This approach may provide a way to obtain a specific aetiological diagnosis without resort to brain biopsy. Empirical antiviral therapy is indicated in patients who develop presumed viral encephalitis in a non-epidemic setting. Without specific antiviral therapy approximately 70% of patients with herpes simplex encephalitis die, and nearly all of the survivors have permanent neurological sequelae. Acyclovir, 10 mg/kg intravenously every eight hours, is the most effective therapeutic agent currently available. Prognosis for survival and recovery of neurological function is much better in patients treated early in the course of the illness; where therapy with acyclovir is instituted before the fifth day of illness the survival rate is approximately 90%.

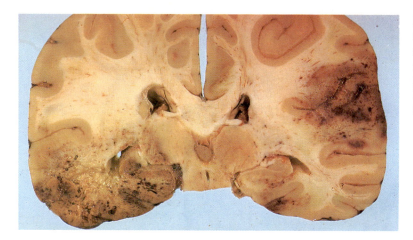

Fig. 5.7 Herpes simplex encephalitis. Coronal brain section showing haemorrhagic necrosis of the cortex and white matter of the right temporal and left parietal lobes. Courtesy of Dr GD Perkin.

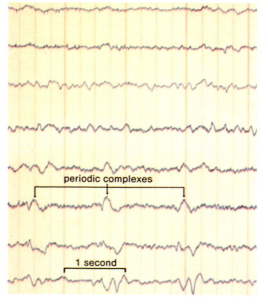

Fig. 5.8 Herpes simplex encephalitis. EEG showing periodic polyphasic complexes every 1½ seconds maximal in the left occipital region.

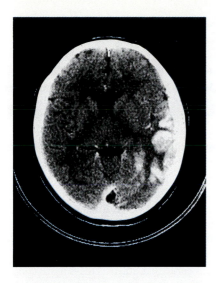

Fig. 5.9 Herpes simplex encephalitis. CT scan done late in the course of the illness, showing enhancement of gyral structures in the left temporal area and adjacent cerebral oedema. Courtesy of Dr J Curé.

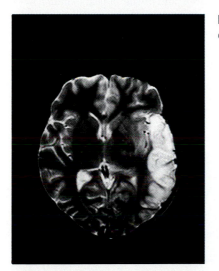

Fig. 5.10 Herpes simplex encephalitis. MRI scan showing extensive involvement of the left temporal area. Courtesy of Dr J Curé.

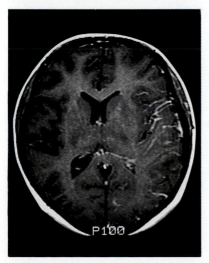

Fig. 5.11 Herpes simplex encephalitis. MRI scan showing enhancement by gadolinium of gyral structures in the left temporal area. Courtesy of Dr J Curé.

VARICELLA-ZOSTER VIRUS

Encephalitis is a rare complication of herpes zoster. It is seen most frequently in the elderly, in association with disseminated or cranial herpes zoster (Fig. 5.15), and in immunocompromised patients, especially those with lymphoproliferative malignancies. Whether the encephalitis is due to direct viral invasion of the CNS, or results from an immunological reaction, is unknown.

Common clinical features include fever, headache, confusion, memory deficit, disorientation and depressed level of consciousness, sometimes progressing to coma. CNS manifestations usually develop about a week after the appearance of skin lesions, and 1–2 days after evidence of dissemination. Untreated, the illness normally lasts approximately 14 days. Most patients recover completely without significant neurological sequelae. Diagnosis is usually made on clinical grounds. Diagnostic criteria include clinical evidence of herpes zoster, encephalopathic state, diffusely abnormal EEG, and CSF abnormalities compatible with encephalitis.

Most patients with herpes zoster encephalitis have a mononuclear pleocytosis and increased protein concentration in the CSF, but up to 40% of those with herpes zoster without encephalitis have abnormalities in the CSF. Varicella-zoster virus (VZV) is rarely isolated from the CSF, but a rise in titre of antibody to VZV may be demonstrated in the CSF in some, but not all patients.

Treatment with high doses of intravenous acyclovir (10 mg/kg every eight hours) intravenously usually results in a rapid and dramatic clinical response, with defervescence and resolution of encephalopathy and EEG abnormalities within 72 hours. Treatment should be continued for approximately one week.

A well-recognized but rare complication of chickenpox is cerebellar ataxia. This is more common in children, and usually appears within a week after the onset of the rash. In addition to ataxia, fever, vertigo, tremor, vomiting and abnormalities of speech may occur. CSF examination usually reveals lymphocytic pleocytosis and elevated concentration of protein. Resolution normally occurs within a few

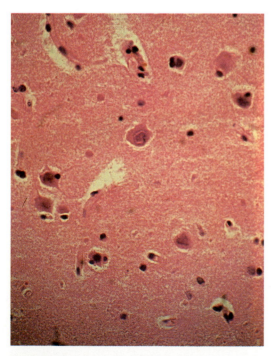

Fig. 5.12 Herpes simplex encephalitis. Intranuclear inclusion in nerve cell. × 250. H&E stain. Courtesy of Professor JE Banatvala.

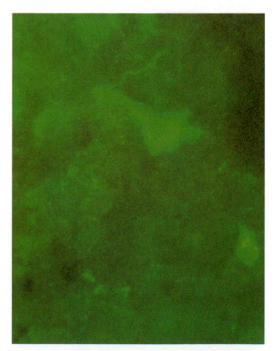

Fig. 5.13 Herpes simplex encephalitis: brain biopsy. The neurons staining bright green are heavily infected with herpes simplex virus. Immunofluorescent preparation. Courtesy of Dr S. Fisher-Hoch.

weeks. A more severe generalized encephalitis may also complicate chickenpox, especially in adults. These patients exhibit fever, severe headache, vomiting, disorientation, depression in the level of consciousness and, frequently, seizures. This type of severe encephalitis typically lasts for several weeks. The case-fatality rate may be as high as 20%, and prominent neurological sequelae occur in a significant proportion of survivors.

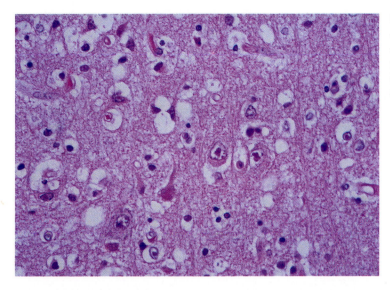

Fig. 5.14 Herpes simplex encephalitis. Lymphocytic infiltration and a characteristic inclusion body at the edge of a necrotic lesion in the brain. H&E section. Courtesy of Dr H Okazaki.

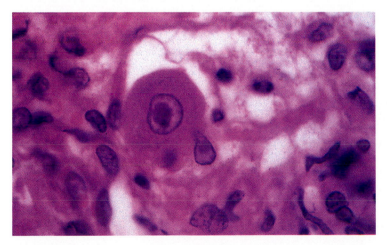

Fig. 5.15 Trigeminal herpes zoster. Cowdry type A inclusions in the nucleus of a ganglion cell and a satellite cell in a patient with Hodgkin's disease. H&E stain. Courtesy of D Toussant and JJ Van de Haeghen, with permission from *Ophthalmologia*.

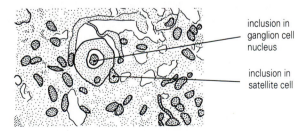

inclusion in ganglion cell nucleus

inclusion in satellite cell

OTHER VIRAL ENCEPHALITIDES

In addition to the agents already discussed, a large number of other viruses may cause encephalitis. Many of these are transmitted to man by arthropods, either mosquitoes or ticks. Some of the more important arthropod-borne encephalitides are listed in Fig. 5.16. Severity of illness and case-fatality rate vary considerably. For example, in eastern equine encephalitis the case fatality rate in man is 50–70%, and up to 70% of survivors may have serious neurological sequelae. Severe illness is also observed commonly in Japanese B encephalitis. In contrast, fatal cases of California encephalitis (La Crosse virus) are extremely rare.

Encephalitis occasionally occurs as a complication of other viral diseases, including mumps, measles, rubella, influenza, enteroviral infections and infectious mononucleosis. A distinct clinical syndrome of chronic meningoencephalitis due to enteroviruses (primarily echoviruses) has been described in immunocompromised people, most commonly in those with X-linked agammaglobulinaemia.

MYCOPLASMA ENCEPHALITIS

Encephalitis or meningoencephalitis, and occasionally other neurological complications, may occur in association with pneumonia due to *Mycoplasma pneumoniae* in up to 10% of cases).

Some Important Arthropod-borne Encephalitides	
Disease	**Geographic Distribution**
Mosquito-borne	
Eastern equine encephalitis	Eastern, Gulf coast and southern USA
Western equine encephalitis	Western and midwestern USA; western Canada
Venezuelan equine encephalitis	South and Central America; southern USA
St. Louis encephalitis	Central, western and southern USA
Japanese B encephalitis	Japan, Korea, Southeast Asia, China, India
California encephalitis (La Crosse virus)	Northern USA
Murray Valley encephalitis	Australia
Rift Valley encephalitis	Eastern and southern Africa
Tick-borne	
Colorado tick fever	Mountains of western USA
Tick-borne encephalitis	Former USSR, Central Europe, Scandinavia
Kyasanur Forest disease	India
Omsk haemorrhagic fever	Siberia

Fig. 5.16 Some important arthropod-borne encephalitides.

Chapter 6

Encephalitis (II)

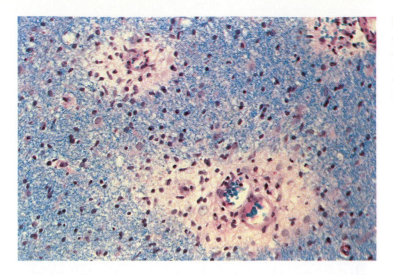

Fig. 6.1 Post-vaccinal encephalomyelitis. Perivascular demyelination and mononuclear inflammation in patient with post-vaccinal encephalomyelitis. Luxol-fast blue stain. Courtesy of Dr P Garen.

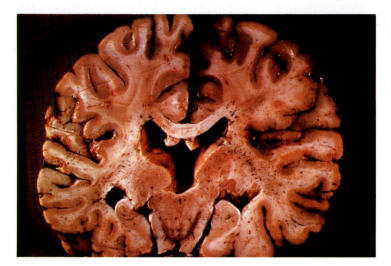

Fig. 6.2 Post-infectious encephalitis. Gross specimen of brain showing multiple punctate haemorrhages and rounded outline of the brain due to cerebral oedema. Courtesy of Dr MJ Wood.

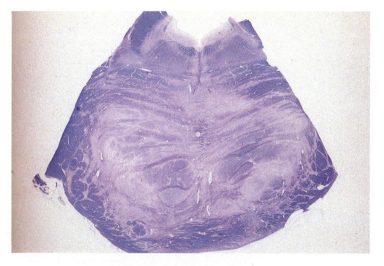

Fig. 6.3 Post-infectious encephalitis. Section of pons showing confluent areas of demyelination. Luxol-fast blue stain. Courtesy of Dr MJ Wood.

POST-INFECTIOUS AND POST-VACCINAL ENCEPHALITIS

Post-infectious and post-vaccinal encephalomyelitis resemble, clinically and pathologically, experimental allergic encephalomyelitis produced by sensitization to central myelin. Indeed, they may be human counterparts of that condition. Post-infectious encephalomyelitis may occur following a wide variety of acute viral infections, including measles, varicella, rubella, mumps and various respiratory infections. Post-vaccinal encephalomyelitis may occur following various immunizations, most commonly following administration of the older neural tissue-derived rabies vaccines. The interval between onset of viral infection or immunization and appearance of symptoms or signs referable to the nervous system is usually 2–12 days. The clinical picture may include evidence of encephalitis or myelitis or both.

Onset of the neurological illness may be relatively abrupt, and seizures and alteration of consciousness are common. The pathological picture is characterized by perivascular infiltration of mononuclear inflammatory cells and perivenous demyelination (Fig. 6.1). In severe cases there may be pronounced cerebral oedema, multiple punctate haemorrhages, and extensive demyelination and necrosis (Figs 6.2, 6.3, 6.4 & 6.5). Examination of the spinal fluid usually reveals elevation in protein concentration and moderate mononuclear pleocytosis. Myelin basic protein may also be present. Prognosis is uncertain, but some patients have made excellent recoveries following long periods of unconsciousness, so vigorous supportive therapy is indicated. Cerebral oedema, seizures, hypoglycaemia and inappropriate secretion of antidiuretic hormone may occur and require specific treatment.

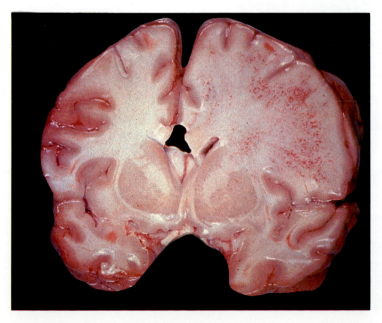

Fig. 6.4 Acute haemorrhagic leucoencephalitis. Coronal brain slice showing swelling of white matter on the right with petechial haemorrhages. Courtesy of Dr GD Perkin.

REYE'S SYNDROME

Reye's syndrome is a disease of unknown aetiology, affecting the liver and central nervous system, which follows a variety of viral infections, most frequently influenza B and varicella. It is seen almost exclusively in children. Typically, nausea and vomiting occur a few days after onset of a viral infection, followed by a change in mental status. Neurological manifestations may include lethargy, delirium, seizures, stupor, coma and respiratory arrest. Hepatomegaly is present, with abnormalities in liver function tests including elevated blood ammonia and prolonged prothrombin time. Jaundice is usually absent. Examination of the cerebrospinal fluid (CSF) reveals normal protein concentration and an

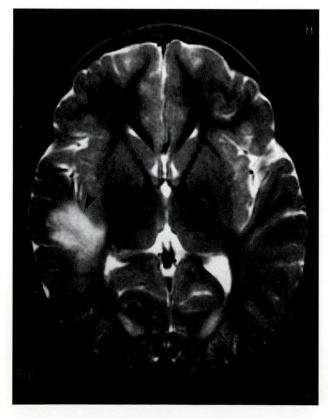

Fig. 6.5 Post-infectious encephalomyelitis. Axial T2-weighted MRI in a child with a history of acute disseminated encephalomyelitis (ADEM). An abnormal hypertense signal is present in the right posterior temporal lobe (arrowhead) and adjacent to the occipital horns (arrows). Courtesy of Dr P Van Tassel.

absence of cells. Histopathological findings in the brain include cerebral oedema and anoxic degeneration of neurons, but little or no inflammation. The lesion in the liver is characterized by fatty infiltration of hepatocytes, with multiple small droplets of lipids uniformly distributed throughout the cells (Fig. 6.6). An extensive recent study revealed an increased incidence of Reye's syndrome in children who have received aspirin for fever resulting from influenza. There is no specific therapy but intensive supportive care including administration of glucose intravenously to correct hypoglycaemia, haemodynamic monitoring, assisted ventilation, and mannitol to lower increased intracranial pressure, may be required. Case-fatality rate ranges from 10–40%, and is highest in children who present in coma.

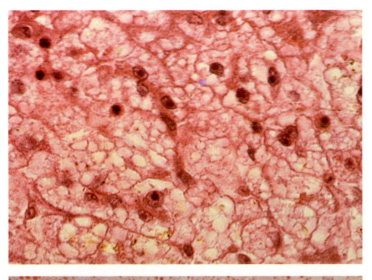
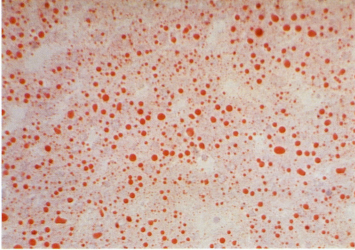

Fig. 6.6 Reye's syndrome. Upper: Section of the liver showing fat droplets in cytoplasmic microvesicles. H&E stain. Lower: Fat globules stained by oil red O.

SLOW VIRAL INFECTIONS

These are progressive neurological diseases caused by transmissible agents, which become manifest only after a very long incubation period of months or years. The transmissible spongiform encephalopathies (Creutzfeldt–Jakob disease, kuru and the Gerstmann–Straussler syndrome) are caused by transmissible agents called prions, which differ markedly from conventional viruses; progressive multifocal leucoencephalopathy and subacute sclerosing panencephalitis are due to more typical viral agents.

The aetiological agents of the transmissible spongiform encephalopathies appear to be very small particles containing little or no nucleic acid. They are highly resistant to a number of physical and chemical agents which inactivate conventional viruses, including various types of radiation, formaldehyde, β-propiolactone, heat and nuclease enzymes. The causative agent of scrapie, a progressive neurological disease of sheep, is the best studied of the slow viruses. Fibrillar or rod-shaped particles, which may be proteins or glycoproteins and are closely associated with cell membranes, have been visualized in the brains of affected animals and humans, and the

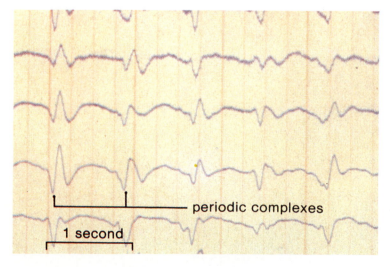

Fig. 6.7 Creutzfeldt–Jakob disease. EEG (position 8) showing periodic complexes at approximately 1.25 Hz.

infectious agent has been partially purified. A 'prion protein' (PrP), mol. wt 27 000–30 000 Da, is present in normal brain tissue, and molecular studies have demonstrated altered forms of PrP in patients with spongiform encephalopathies.

Creutzfeldt–Jakob Disease

Creutzfeldt–Jakob disease is an uncommon progressive cerebral disease characterized by dementia, ataxia and diffuse myoclonic jerking. In most patients dementia becomes profound within six months and death occurs normally within a year of the onset of symptoms. The diagnosis is primarily clinical, but relatively characteristic EEG findings occur at some stage of the illness in more than half of the patients (Fig. 6.7). The CSF is usually normal, although a slight elevation in protein concentration is observed occasionally. CT scanning and MRI often show no abnormalities. Typical neuropathological findings include diffuse loss of neurons, intense proliferation of fibrillary astrocytes (Fig. 6.8) with fibrous gliosis and intracytoplasmic vacuolation, and swelling of both neuronal and astroglial processes,

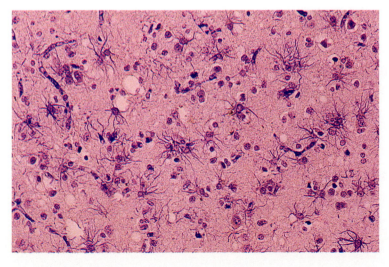

Fig. 6.8 Creutzfeldt–Jakob disease. Loss of neurons, increase in the size of vacuoles (status spongiosus) and proliferation of fibrillary astrocytes. Holzer stain. Courtesy of Dr H Okazaki and Dr B Scheithauer.

resulting in the 'spongy' state (Figs 6.9 & 6.10). In a few patients PAS-positive, amyloid-like plaques are found. In the majority of cases the changes are most severe in the frontal lobes. Creutzfeldt–Jakob disease is worldwide in distribution, with an overall annual incidence of approximately one case per million population. A strikingly increased incidence has been observed in Libyan Jews living in Israel, possibly associated with the eating of animal brains or sheep eyeballs. Sporadic cases have apparently been acquired via person-to-person transmission following neurosurgical procedures, and via administration of a growth hormone made from bovine pituitary glands. Approximately 15% of cases are familial, in a pattern which suggests autosomal dominant transmission.

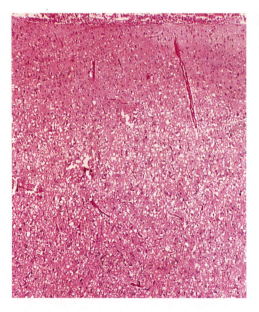

Fig. 6.9 Creutzfeldt–Jakob disease. Histological section of cerebral cortex at low magnification showing multiple vacuoles . Courtesy of Dr H Whitwell.

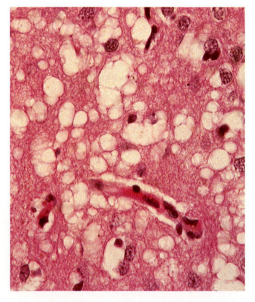

Fig. 6.10 Creutzfeldt–Jakob disease. High power view. Courtesy of Dr H Whitwell.

Kuru

Kuru, which is similar to Creutzfeldt–Jakob disease, is seen only in the highlands of eastern New Guinea, primarily among tribes of the Fore linguistic group. It is characterized by insidious onset of cerebellar ataxia of gait and limbs, with shivering, dysarthria, pyramidal and extrapyramidal signs, involuntary movements and mood changes with eventual development of dementia, dysphagia and ventilatory failure. Neuropathological changes are similar to those of Creutzfeldt–Jakob disease, but are most severe in the cerebellum, and the majority of patients exhibit PAS-positive, amyloid-like plaques. Transmission of kuru apparently occurs during ritual cannibalism of dead kinsmen, probably via cuts on the hands sustained during removal of the brains. Cessation of the practice of ritualistic cannibalism has apparently eliminated transmission of kuru.

Gertsmann–Straussler Syndrome

Gertsmann–Straussler syndrome is an adult-onset, chronic cerebellar ataxia, which is usually familial. Dementia often develops late in the course of the disease. Recent investigations of families with the Gerstmann–Straussler syndrome and other dementing and ataxic illnesses have demonstrated that dementia associated with the abnormal PrP gene may be present in individuals who lack the characteristic neuropathological changes. Neurological disease associated with transmissible prion proteins may be more diverse and more frequent than previously suspected.

Progressive Multifocal Leucoencephalopathy

Progressive multifocal leucoencephalopathy (PML) is a rare, subacute, progressive demyelinating disease of the CNS which occurs almost exclusively in immunocompromised patients. The most common underlying conditions are Hodgkin's disease, chronic lymphocytic leukaemia and AIDS, although a few cases have occurred following renal transplantation. The distribution of PML is worldwide. The causative agent is the JC virus, a member of the polyoma group of papovaviruses. Approximately 75% of adults have antibody to this virus, so PML probably represents the reactivation of a pre-existing latent infection. The characteristic neuropathological finding is focal destruction of myelin (Figs 6.11 & 6.12), with relative preservation of axons. As the disease

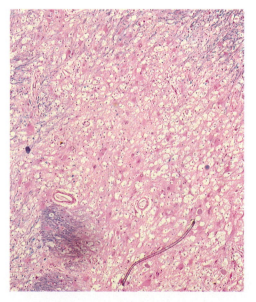

Fig. 6.11 Progressive multifocal leucoencephalopathy. Histological section showing a focus of demyelination, reactive astrocytosis and lipid-laden macrophages. Luxol-fast blue stain. Courtesy of Dr MJ Wood.

progresses the foci of demyelination become confluent, producing large plaques (Figs 6.13 & 6.14). There is little or no inflammatory response. Giant astrocytes, with pleomorphic, hyperchromatic nuclei, sometimes with mitotic figures, indistinguishable from the malignant astrocytes seen in glioblastomas, are often present (Fig. 6.15); these cells may reflect the oncogenic potential of the polyoma virus. Viral particles, 28–40 nm in diameter, may sometimes be seen in the nuclei of oligodendrocytes within the lesions (Figs 6.16, 6.17, 6.18 & 6.19).

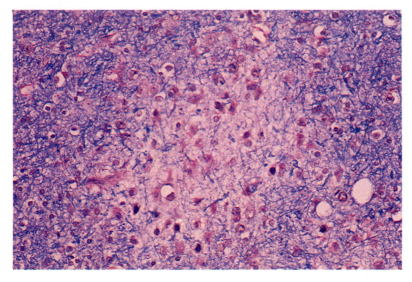

Fig. 6.12 Progressive multifocal leucoencephalopathy. Small focus of demyelination and infiltration by macrophages. Luxol-fast blue–PAS–haematoxylin stain. Courtesy of Dr H Okazaki and Dr B Scheithauer

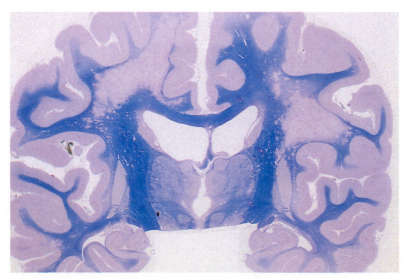

Fig. 6.13 Progressive multifocal leucoencephalopathy. Gross specimen showing confluent zones of demyelination. Luxol-fast blue–cresyl violet stain. Courtesy of Dr H Okazaki and Dr B Scheithauer

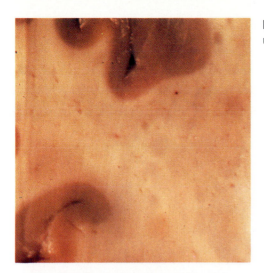

Fig. 6.14 Progressive multifocal leucoencephalopathy. Diffuse white matter loss with focal granular necrosis. Courtesy of Dr P Garen.

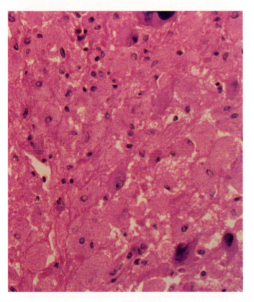

Fig. 6.15 Progressive multifocal leucoencephalopathy. Affected region of white matter displaying numerous background foamy macrophages and bizarre astrocytes with enlarged, hyperchromatic and lobulated nuclei. H&E stain. Courtesy of Dr P Garen.

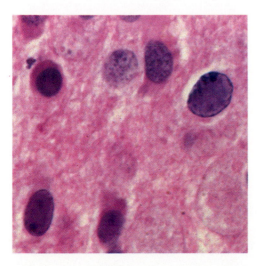

Fig. 6.16 Progressive multifocal leucoencephalopathy. Enlarged oligodendroglial nuclei with homogenous basophilic intranuclear viral inclusions. H&E stain. Courtesy of Dr P Garen.

The illness usually develops rapidly, with death occurring within a few months after appearance of the first neurological symptoms. The clinical findings are diverse, depending on the location of foci of demyelination. Monoparesis, hemiparesis, ataxia, dysarthria, dysphagia, cortical blindness, personality change and mental impairment occur frequently; in the late stage of the disease extensive paralysis, severe dementia and coma may appear. CT scanning and MRI may be useful in localizing the lesions (Figs 6.20 & 6.21); the lesions of PML do not exhibit enhancement on CT scanning, which may help distinguish them from the lesions of toxoplasmosis. The CSF is usually normal. At present there is no effective treatment.

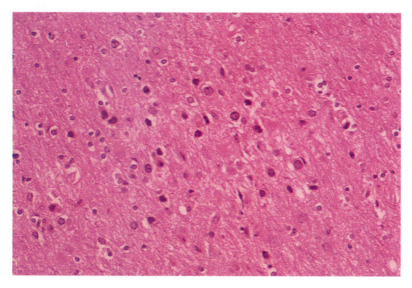

Fig. 6.17 Progressive multifocal leucoencephalopathy. Small focal lesion showing oligodendroglial nuclei filled with amphophilic inclusion bodies. H&E stain. Courtesy of Dr H Okazaki and Dr B Scheithauer

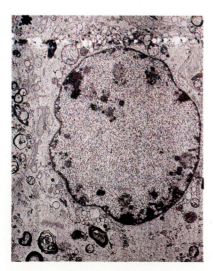

Fig. 6.18 Progressive multifocal leucoencephalopathy. Electron micrograph showing oligodendrocyte nucleus containing diffuse intranuclear viral particles of JC virus. Courtesy of Dr P Garen.

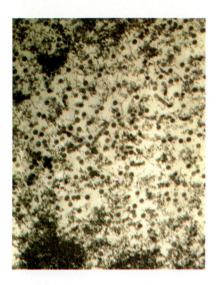

Fig. 6.19 Progressive multifocal leucoencephalopathy. Higher power electron micrograph demonstrating round and filamentous papovavirus particles. Courtesy of Dr P Garen.

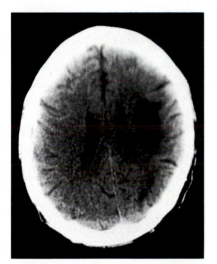

Fig. 6.20 Progressive multifocal leucoencephalopathy. CT scan showing a large hypodense lesion in the left parietal region. Courtesy of Dr J Curé.

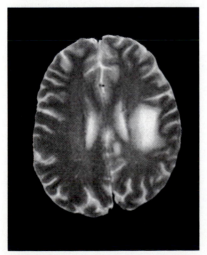

Fig. 6.21 Progressive multifocal leucoencephalopathy. MRI scan of same patient showing a large lesion in the left parietal region and a smaller lesion close to the midline. Courtesy of Dr J Curé.

Subacute Sclerosing Panencephalitis

Subacute sclerosing panencephalitis (SSPE) is a progressive inflammatory neurological disease of children and adolescents which is related to infection with the measles virus. Patients with SSPE have in their brains large amounts of a defective form of the measles virus, which can be cultivated only with difficulty in certain susceptible cell lines. The SSPE virus may represent a variant of the measles virus resulting from mutation, or the result of a recombination between the measles virus and some other viral agent. It has been suggested that the host immune response may be more important in the causation of SSPE than the viral infection itself. High levels of measles antibody might damage virus-infected cells, or sensitized lymphocytes might be cytotoxic to infected target cells.

SSPE is a subacute encephalitis involving grey and white matter of both cerebral hemispheres and brainstem, with perivascular and diffuse infiltrates of lymphocytes and plasma cells (Fig. 6.22). As the disease progresses there is destruction of neurons, diffuse proliferation of glial cells and degeneration of myelin (Fig. 6.23). Eosinophilic intranuclear inclusion bodies with surrounding halos (Cowdry type A inclusions) are seen in glial cells and neurons (Figs 6.24, 6.25 & 6.26). By electron microscopy the inclusions are seen to contain tubular paramyxovirus-like nuclear capsids, 17–19 nm in diameter; these inclusion bodies stain specifically with anti-measles virus antibody. SSPE usually appears approximately seven years after clinical measles; the disease very rarely follows measles immunization. Widespread immunization against measles in the USA and other countries has resulted in a dramatic fall in the incidence of SSPE. The average age of onset is between seven and eight years. The first stage of the illness is characterized by poor school performance, intellectual decline and abnormal behaviour, often diagnosed as a psychological problem. Weeks or months later, more severe intellectual deterioration, seizures, myoclonic jerks and apraxia may appear. Eventually rigidity, hyperactive reflexes, extensor plantar responses and a decorticate state ensue. Death usually occurs after a few months or years; progression is more rapid in children. A characteristic finding in the CSF is increased IgG with oligoclonal bands exhibiting measles antibody activity; these are not found in patients with measles. Titres of measles antibody in serum and CSF may continue to rise throughout the course of the illness. A radionuclide brain scan and CT scans may show the location and extent of the lesions, and relatively characteristic EEG abnormalities have been described. There is no effective treatment for SSPE at the present time.

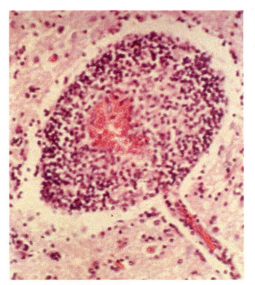

Fig. 6.22 Subacute sclerosing panencephalitis. Very intense perivascular mononuclear inflammatory exudate, with subtle migration of inflammatory cells into the surrounding cerebral cortex. H&E stain.

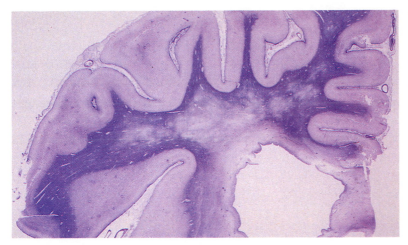

Fig. 6.23 Subacute sclerosing panencephalitis. Gross specimen showing marked fibrous astrocytosis in the frontal white matter. Holzer glial fibril stain. Courtesy of Dr H Okazaki and Dr B Scheithauer.

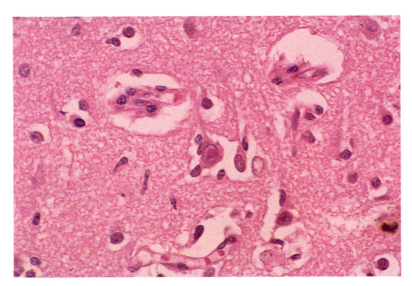

Fig. 6.24 Subacute sclerosing panencephalitis. Multiple eosinophilic intracytoplasmic inclusions in neurons. H&E stain. Courtesy of Dr H Okazaki and Dr B Scheithauer.

Fig. 6.25 Subacute sclerosing panencephalitis. Eosinophilic intranuclear inclusion bodies composed of RNA and ribonuclear protein. Luxol-fast blue and H&E stains.

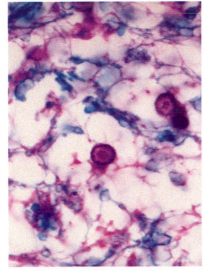

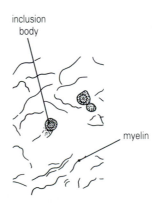

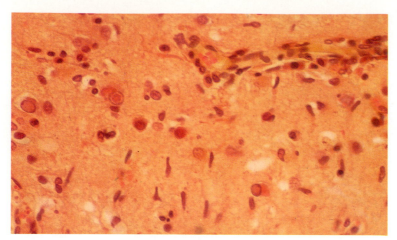

Fig. 6.26 Subacute sclerosing panencephalitis. Upper: Cortex showing an intranuclear inclusion body and perivascular lymphocytic cuffing. Haematoxylin and Van Gieson's stain. × 500.
Lower: A high power view of an inclusion body. Lendrum's phloxine tartrazine stain. × 1500. Courtesy of Dr GD Perkin.

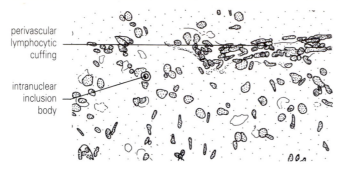

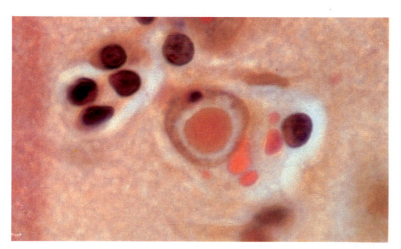

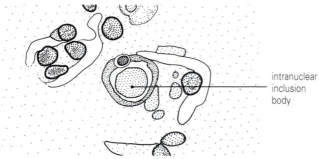

Chapter 7

Brain Abscess and Related Infections

BRAIN ABSCESS

Bacterial Brain Abscess

Bacterial abscess of the brain may arise by direct extension from a contiguous focus of infection, by the haematogenous route, following trauma, or may be unassociated with any overt underlying cause (cryptogenic abscess). The most common mechanism of spread is from a contiguous focus, usually sinusitis or otitis media, and the frontal and temporal lobes are the most common sites of brain abscess. Haematogenous spread can occur from any site of primary infection, but is most commonly associated with infections within the chest, including lung abscess, bronchiectasis and empyema. Head trauma associated with brain abscess includes skull fracture, neurosurgical procedures, pencil tip injuries to the eye in children and lawn dart injuries to the head. Many cryptogenic brain abscesses probably originate as dental infections. Two other conditions associated with a very high incidence of brain abscess are hereditary haemorrhagic telangiectasia with pulmonary arteriovenous malformations, and cyanotic congenital heart disease (Fig. 7.1). In both conditions the normal pulmonary capillary filter is bypassed, and in cyanotic congenital heart disease the polycythaemia and reduced brain capillary blood flow may lead to reduced tissue oxygenation and microinfarction. In the early or 'cerebritis' stage of brain abscess there is no definite capsule around the area of necrosis (Figs 7.2 & 7.3), but after about ten days a capsule forms around the abscess cavity (Figs 7.4, 7.5 & 7.6). Eventually, the inflammatory

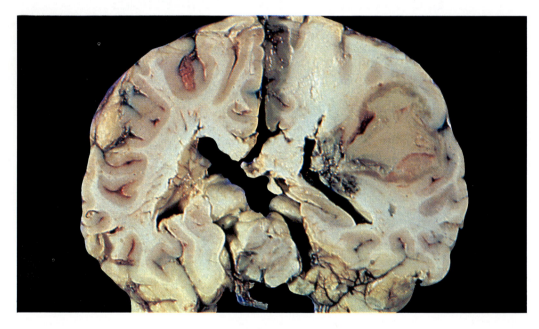

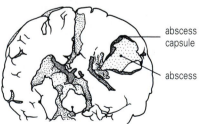

Fig. 7.1 Cerebral abscess. Abscess in the right cerebral hemisphere. This 24-year-old man had Fallot's tetralogy. He gave a history of right-sided headache over three weeks. There were no abnormal neurological findings. The patient died 24 hours after admission. Courtesy of Dr M Gawel.

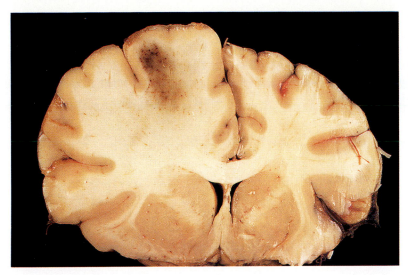

Fig. 7.2 Brain abscess. Gross specimen showing an area of early infection with inflammatory reaction but no tissue liquefaction (cerebritis) in the left frontal lobe. Courtesy of Dr H Okazaki and Dr B Scheithauer.

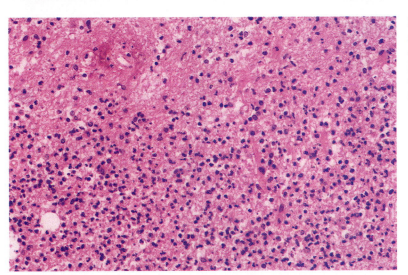

Fig. 7.3 Brain abscess. Microscopic section showing cerebritis without tissue liquefaction. H&E stain. Courtesy of Dr H Okazaki and Dr B Scheithauer.

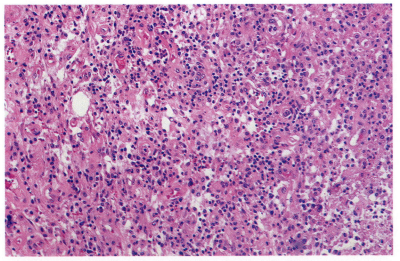

Fig. 7.4 Brain abscess. A zone of intense capillary proliferation and acute inflammatory cell infiltration (inflammatory granulation tissue) adjacent to an abscess cavity. H&E stain. Courtesy of Dr H Okazaki and Dr B Scheithauer.

lation tissue matures into a thick collagenous wall, which prevents further extension of the infection (Fig. 7.7). The wall may be strong enough to allow total surgical excision of the abscess without spilling its contents (Fig. 7.8). Anaerobic and microaerophilic bacteria are commonly isolated from brain abscesses (Figs 7.9 & 7.10). The most common organisms encountered are microaerophilic streptococci of the *S. milleri* group, *Bacteroides* species, members of the Enterobacteriaceae and *Staphylococcus aureus*. Occasionally, *Actinomyces israelii* is isolated (Figs 7.11 & 7.12).

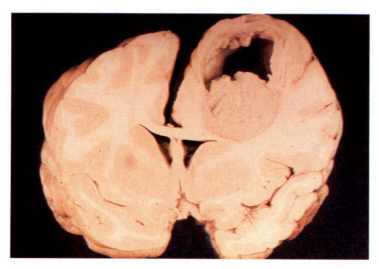

Fig. 7.5 Brain abscess. Coronal section revealing chronic brain abscess due to *Staphylococcus aureus* in the left frontal lobe in a 16-year-old girl. The border of the abscess cavity reveals a linear region of brownish discolouration which represents the capsule of the abscess.

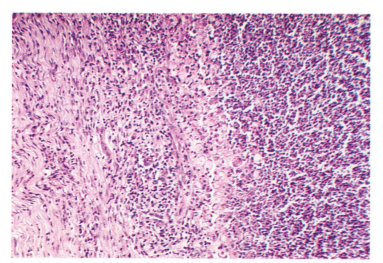

Fig. 7.6 Brain abscess. Histological section of a chronic brain abscess due to *Staphylococcus aureus*. At the centre is an acute inflammatory exudate bordered by zones of macrophages, lymphocytes and plasma cells. Outside this is the layer of fibrosis in the collagenous capsule. H&E stain.

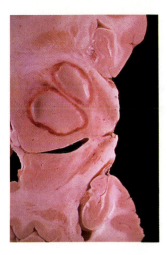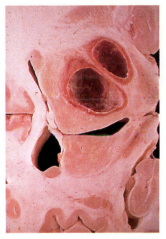

Fig. 7.7 Brain abscess. Gross specimen showing two well-encapsulated abscesses, before (left) and after (right) removal of pus from the abscess cavities. Courtesy of Dr H Okazaki and Dr B Scheithauer.

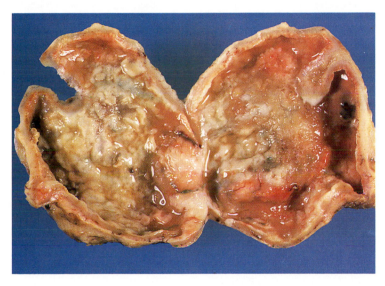

Fig. 7.8 Brain abscess. Surgical specimen showing tough, thick wall which allowed removal of the abscess without spilling its contents. Courtesy of Dr H Okazaki and Dr B Scheithauer.

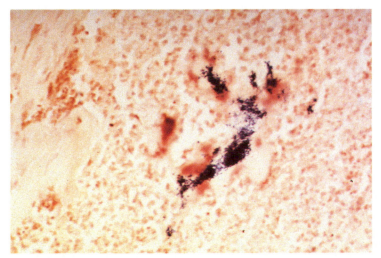

Fig. 7.9 Brain abscess. Histological section of necrotic brain tissue. Clumps of Gram-positive bacteria can be seen within the necrotic material. Brown and Brenn stain. Courtesy of Dr JR Cantey.

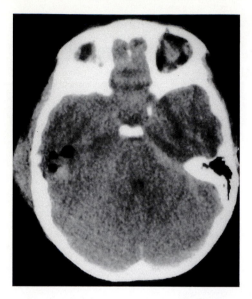

Fig. 7.10 Brain abscess due to *Clostridium perfringens*. CT scan showing gas formation in the lesion in the right parietal area and oedema of extracranial tissue. Courtesy of Dr MJ Wood.

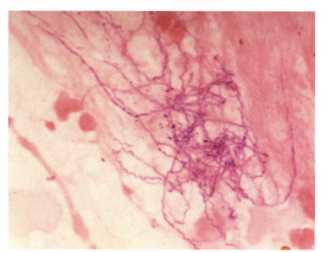

Fig. 7.11 Brain abscess. *Actinomyces israelii*, filamentous Gram-positive bacilli, within inflammatory exudate. Gram's stain. Courtesy of Dr JF John, Jr.

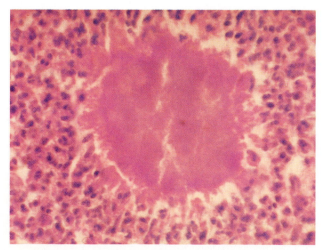

Fig. 7.12 Brain abscess. 'Sulphur granule' in necrotic inflammatory exudate in a cerebellar abscess due to *Actinomyces israelii*. H&E stain.

Fungal Brain Abscess

Brain abscesses due to fungi are seen primarily in immunocompromised patients. In infections due to *Candida albicans* the characteristic lesion is a microabscess (Figs 7.13 & 7.14). Especially in patients with severe burns, these microabscesses may be extremely abundant (Fig. 7.15). The fungi are best demonstrated by silver stain (Fig. 7.16) or by the periodic acid–Schiff technique. Invasive aspergillosis can cause multiple brain abscesses (Figs 7.17 & 7.18). Extensive invasion of blood vessel walls (Fig. 7.19) is characteristic. The large branching hyphae are easily demonstrated with silver stains (Figs 7.20 & 7.21). Occasionally, invasion of the wall of a major cerebral vessel results in massive haemorrhagic

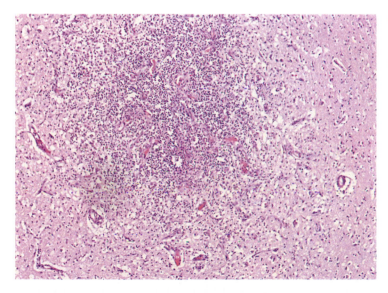

Fig. 7.13 *Candida* brain abscess. Focal acute cerebritis with acute inflammation caused by *Candida* H&E stain. Courtesy of Dr P Garen.

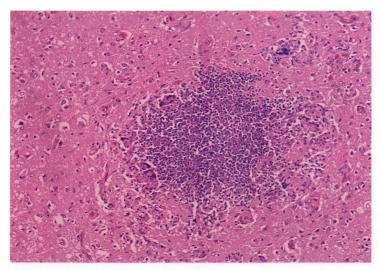

Fig. 7.14 *Candida* brain abscess. Microabscess consisting of a small central collection of pus cells surrounded by a zone of granulomatous cellular reaction with giant cells. H&E stain. Courtesy of Dr H Okazaki and Dr B Scheithauer.

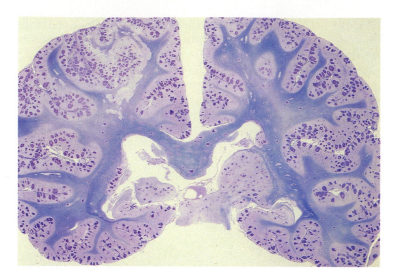

Fig. 7.15 *Candida* brain abscess. Numerous, mainly cortical, lesions in the cerebral hemispheres in a young girl with extensive burns. Luxol-fast blue–cresyl violet stain. Courtesy of Dr H Okazaki and Dr B Scheithauer.

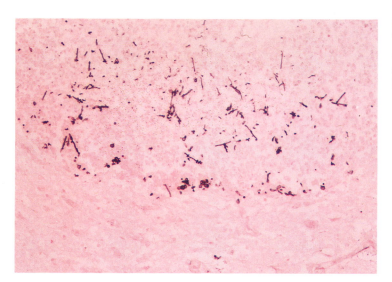

Fig 7.16 *Candida* brain abscess. Yeast and pseudohyphae of *Candida albicans* demonstrated by a silver stain. Courtesy of Dr H Okazaki and Dr B Scheithauer.

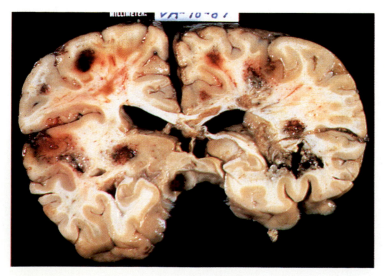

Fig. 7.17 Aspergillosis. Multiple haemorrhagic areas of acute necrosis present in both cerebral hemispheres. Courtesy of Dr P Garen.

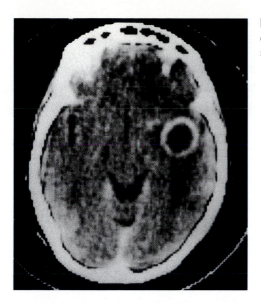

Fig. 7.18 Brain abscess due to *Aspergillus*. CT scan showing a large abscess cavity surrounded by a thick rim in the left temporal area, and a smaller lesion in the right parietal area. Courtesy of Dr MJ Wood.

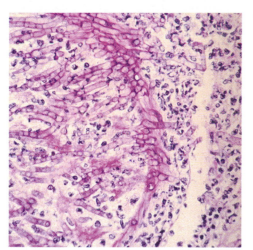

Fig. 7.19 Cerebral aspergillosis. Numerous septate hyphae invading a blood vessel wall associated with acute and chronic inflammatory reaction. Periodic acid–Schiff stain.

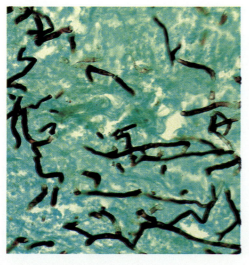

Fig. 7.20 Aspergillosis. *Aspergillus* hyphae with dichotomous branching and septae. Gomori methenamine silver stain. Courtesy of Dr P Garen.

infarction which is rapidly fatal (Fig. 7.22). Rhinocerebral mucormycosis, due to zygomycetes such as rhizopus and mucor, is seen mainly but not exclusively in patients with uncontrolled diabetes mellitus. It begins with infection of the oral and nasal mucous membranes and paranasal sinuses (Figs 7.23, 7.24, 7.25 & 7.26), and extends through the tissues, including bone, to reach the brain (Fig. 7.27). Invasion of the orbit may cause facial and ocular pain, proptosis and ophthalmoplegia, followed

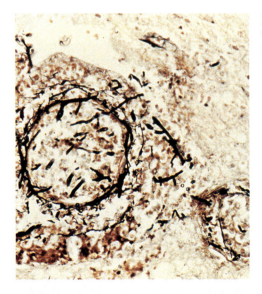

Fig. 7.21 Aspergillosis. *Aspergillus* hyphae ensnared in vascular thrombi. Hyphae permeate adjacent vascular wall and invade brain parenchyma. Gomori methenamine silver stain. Courtesy of Dr P Garen.

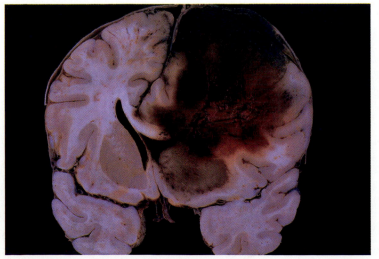

Fig. 7.22 Aspergillosis. Gross specimen showing massive haemorrhagic infarction of the right cerebral hemisphere due to infection of the wall of a large artery. Courtesy of Dr H Okazaki and Dr B Scheithauer.

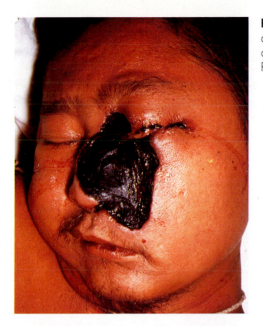

Fig. 7.23 Rhinocerebral mucormycosis. Advanced case with necrosis of nasal and maxillary tissue and black eschar. Note the periorbital oedema and serosanguinous discharge from the eye. Courtesy of Professor RY Cartwright.

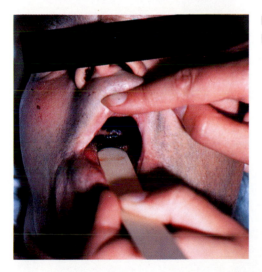

Fig. 7.24 Rhinocerebral mucormycosis with infarction of the hard palate. Courtesy of Dr J Snape.

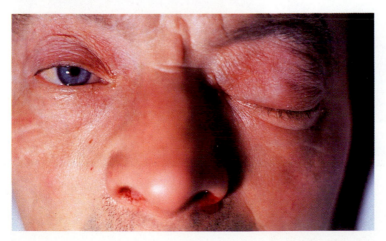

Fig. 7.25 Rhinocerebral mucormycosis. Bloodstained nasal discharge with left-sided ptosis and proptosis. Courtesy of Dr J Innes.

by evidence of arterial or retro-orbital venous occlusion (Fig. 7.28). Thrombosis of the internal carotid artery, with contralateral hemiplegia, may occur. The organism can be found in culture (Fig. 7.29) and biopsy material (Figs 7.30 & 7.31). There is extensive invasion of vascular structures (Figs 7.32 & 7.33) and massive necrosis of brain tissue (Figs 7.34, 7.35, 7.36 & 7.37).

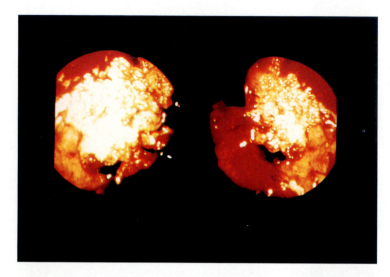

Fig. 7.26 Rhinocerebral mucormycosis. View through nasal speculum showing fungal material arising from nasal turbinates. Courtesy of Professor RY Cartwright.

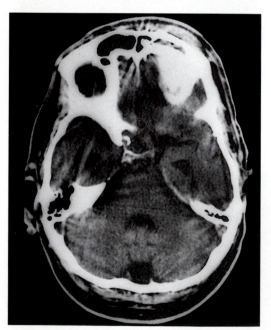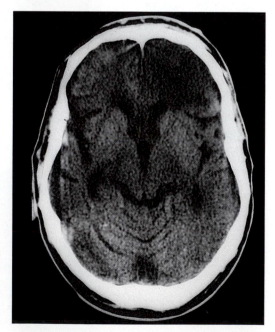

Fig. 7.27 Rhinocerebral mucormycosis. Immunosuppressed patient with acute myelomonocytic leukaemia and rhinocerebral mucormycosis. Left: Non-contrast axial CT scan showing partial opacification of the left frontal sinus and soft tissue thickening in the subcutaneous tissues of the left forehead. Right: A higher section, revealing acute left frontal infarct secondary to vascular occlusion by the fungus. Courtesy of Dr P Van Tassel.

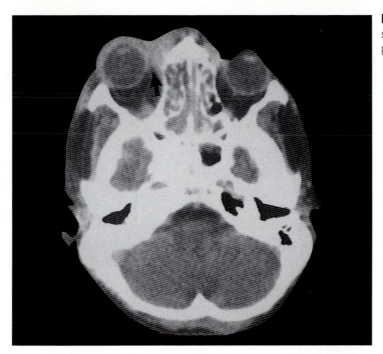

Fig. 7.28 Mucormycosis. CT scan showing a periorbital mass (arrow) with proptosis. Courtesy of Dr GD Perkin.

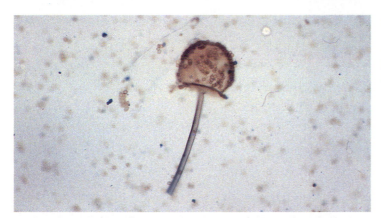

Fig. 7.29 Rhinocerebral mucormycosis. Sporangiospore of *Rhizopus oryzae* (family Mucoraceae) isolated from the patient in Fig. 7.24. Courtesy of Dr J Innes.

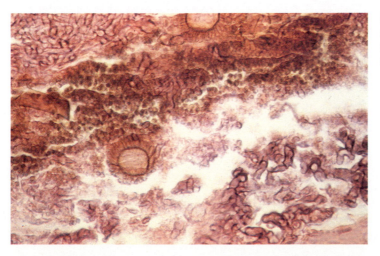

Fig. 7.30 Rhinocerebral mucormycosis. Mucor organisms visible in biopsy, showing irregular branching hyphae and sporangia. Courtesy of Professor RY Cartwright.

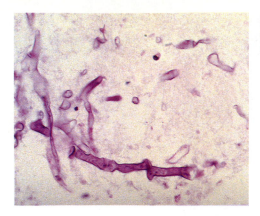

Fig. 7.31 Rhinocerebral mucormycosis. Brain biopsy from a diabetic patient showing the large non-septate hyphae. Periodic acid–Schiff stain.

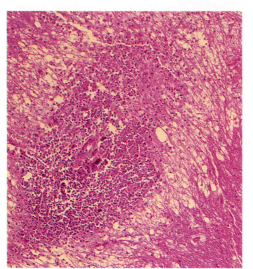

Fig. 7.32 Rhinocerebral mucormycosis. Vessel obstruction by mucor resulting in focal perivascular acute necrosis. H&E stain. Courtesy of Dr P Garen.

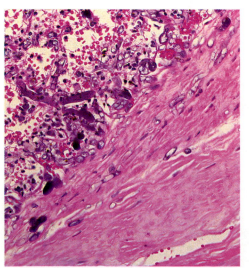

Fig. 7.33 Rhinocerebral mucormycosis. Wall of thrombosed internal carotid artery with hyphae of mucor present in thrombus and arterial wall. H&E stain. Courtesy of Dr P Garen.

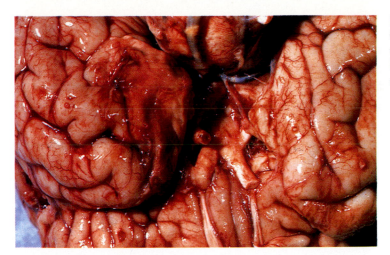

Fig. 7.34 Rhinocerebral mucormycosis. Gross brain specimen viewed from base with acute superficial necrosis of temporal lobe and thrombosis of left internal carotid artery. Courtesy of Dr P Garen.

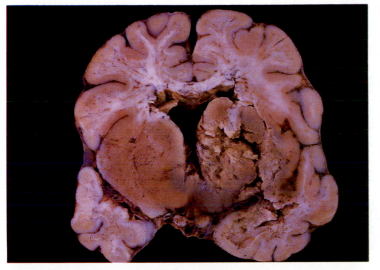

Fig. 7.35 Rhinocerebral mucormycosis. Gross specimen showing extensive infarction of the orbital surface of the frontal lobes and adjacent temporal lobes and basal ganglia due to fungal invasion of the walls of major blood vessels. Courtesy of Dr H Okazaki and Dr B Scheithauer.

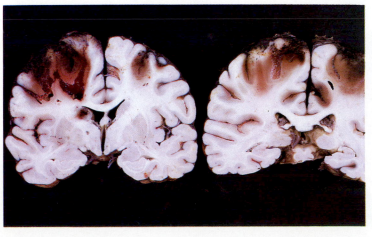

Fig. 7.36 Mucormycosis. Gross specimen showing haemorrhagic infarction of the brain due to haematogenous spread of mucormycosis from the lung. Courtesy of Dr H Okazaki and Dr B Scheithauer.

Other Causes of Brain Abscess

Other causes of brain abscess in immunocompromised patients are *Listeria monocytogenes* (Fig. 7.38) and *Nocardia asteroides* (Figs 7.39, 7.40 & 7.41), the latter usually in association with pulmonary infection (Fig. 7.42). Patients with AIDS also have an increased incidence of brain abscess due to *Toxoplasma gondii* (see Chapter 9), *Cryptococcus neoformans*, *Mycobacterium* species, and *Salmonella* group B. In certain areas of the world parasites such as *Entamoeba histolytica*, *Schistosoma japonicum* (Fig. 7.43),

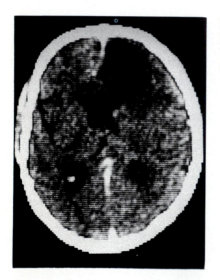

Fig. 7.37 Rhinocerebral mucormycosis. CT scan showing a large necrotic mass lesion in the left frontal lobe displacing the falx cerebri and inferior sagittal sinus. The ventricular system in the area is also distorted and displaced. Courtesy of Dr GD Hungerford.

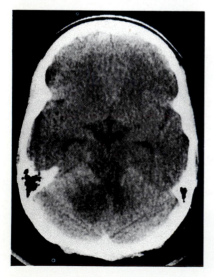

Fig. 7.38 *Listeria monocytogenes* rhombencephalitis. CT scan showing oedema (extensive hypodense lesion) involving brain stem structures. There is obliteration of perimesencephalic cisterns and effacement of the aqueduct of Sylvius, producing early dilatation of the temporal horns of the lateral ventricles. Courtesy of Dr MJ Wood.

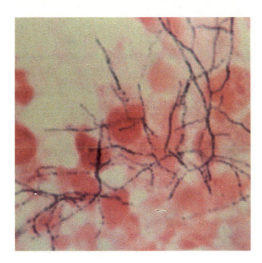

Fig. 7.39 Nocardiosis. In this pus smear *Nocardia asteroides* appears mainly as irregularly staining filaments, but a variety of forms is often seen, including rods, cocci and even spiral forms. Courtesy of AE Prevost.

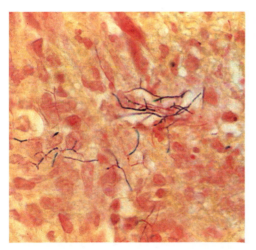

Fig. 7.40 Nocardiosis. Brain abscess revealing filamentous Gram-positive bacilli of *Nocardia asteroides*. Brown and Brenn stain. Courtesy of Dr P Garen.

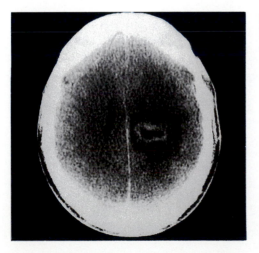

Fig. 7.41 Brain abscess due to *Nocardia*. CT scan showing a single hypodense lesion surrounded by a thin rim and an extensive area of oedema in the left parietal region. Courtesy of Dr MJ Wood.

Paragonimus westermani, Echinococcus granulosus (Figs 7.44, 7.45, 7.46, 7.47 & 7.48) and *Cysticercus cellulosae* (see Chapter 9) are relatively common causes of brain abscess. Focal lesions of the brain may also be seen occasionally in Whipple's disease (Fig. 7.49).

Clinical Presentation and Diagnosis of Brain Abscess

The clinical picture of brain abscess is highly variable. The illness usually develops more gradually than that associated with pyogenic meningitis, but 75% of patients seek medical attention within two

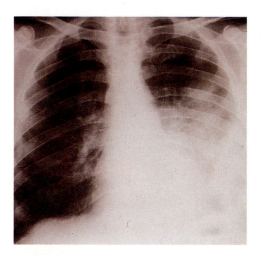

Fig. 7.42 Pulmonary nocardiasis. Radiograph showing consolidation in the lower lobe of the left lung and associated pleural effusion.

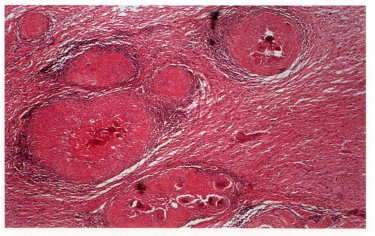

Fig. 7.43 Schistosomiasis. Eggs of *Schistosoma japonicum* in gliotic brain with surrounding macrophage and chronic inflammatory cell response. H&E stain.

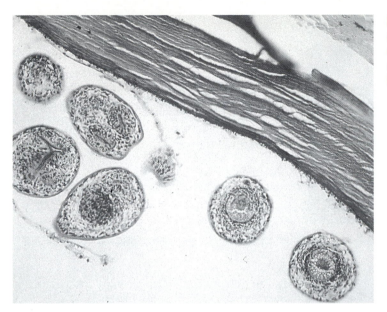

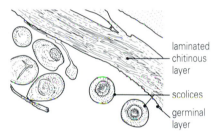

laminated
chitinous
layer

scolices

germinal
layer

Fig. 7.44 Hydatid disease. Wall of cyst with laminated chitinous layer and inner germinal layer, surrounding scolices with invaginated heads. Courtesy of Dr GD Perkin.

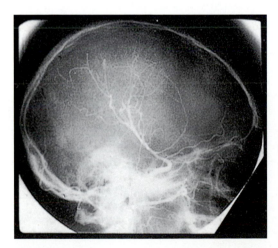

Fig. 7.45 Echinococcosis. Cerebral angiography showing displacement of vessels by a large mass in the frontal region. Courtesy of Dr H Whitwell.

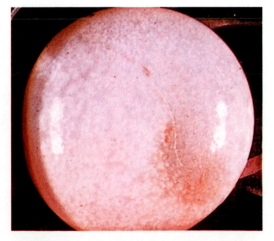

Fig. 7.46 Echinococcosis. Cyst removed from patient in Fig. 7.45. Courtesy of Dr H Whitwell.

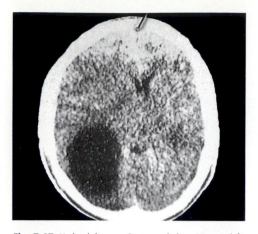

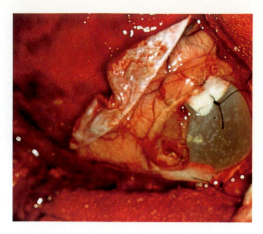

Fig. 7.47 Hydatid disease. Cyst revealed on CT scan (left) and at craniotomy (right). Courtesy of Dr A Ameen.

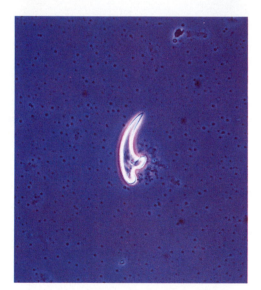

Fig. 7.48 Echinococcosis. Fluid from cyst viewed under polarized light showing hook of hydatid. Courtesy of Dr H Whitwell.

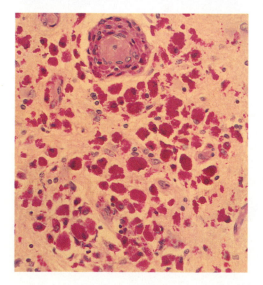

Fig. 7.49 Whipple's disease. Section of brain showing a focal lesion with many PAS-positive macrophages surrounding a small blood vessel. PAS stain. Courtesy of Dr P Garen.

weeks of the onset of symptoms. The classic triad of fever, headache and focal neurological deficits is seen in less than 50% of patients. Severe progressive headache is the most common presenting symptom. Nausea and vomiting, seizures and altered mental status are also relatively common.

Lumbar puncture is contraindicated; findings in the CSF are not often helpful in the diagnosis and the procedure is dangerous because of the risk of herniation. CT scanning has revolutionized the diagnosis, therapy and prognosis of brain abscess. The CT scan yields evidence of brain abscess in approximately 95% of patients beyond the stage of cerebri-

tis, and provides more accurate localization of the lesion(s) than the studies that were previously available. The characteristic appearance is a hypodense centre bounded by a uniform ring of enhancement, which is surrounded by a variable hypodense region of oedema (Figs 7.50, 7.51, 7.52 & 7.53). Technetium-99 brain scanning and MRI may be slightly more sensitive than CT scanning during the cerebritis stage of infection. Occasionally it may be difficult to differentiate between brain abscess and a necrotic tumour; the addition of an Indium–111 radionuclide scan to the CT scan may help distinguish inflammatory from neoplastic lesions.

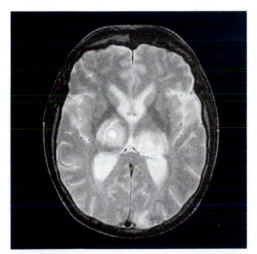

Fig. 7.50 Brain abscess. MRI scan showing bilateral abscess cavities in the region of the basal ganglia. Courtesy of Dr J Curé.

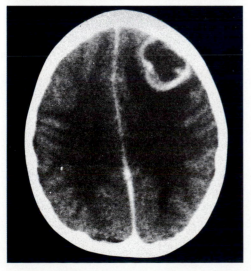

Fig. 7.51 Brain abscess. CT scan showing the typical appearance of a brain abscess in the left frontal lobe with enhancement of the capsule. The uniform thin wall is characteristic of abscess rather than tumour. Courtesy of Dr GD Hungerford.

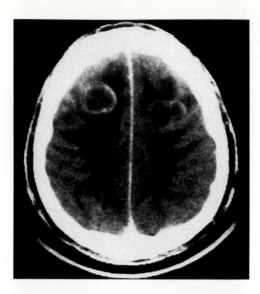

Fig. 7.52 Brain abscess. CT scan showing multiple brain lesions as abscesses in the frontal lobes, with enhancement of the capsule of the abscess. Courtesy of Dr H Okazaki and Dr B Scheithauer.

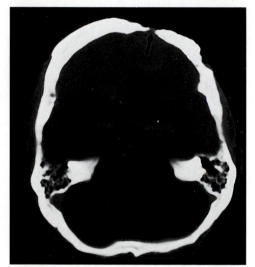

Fig. 7.53 Brain abscess. Upper: CT scan in a patient with multiple surgeries for basal cell carcinomas on the forehead, showing a dehiscent left frontal bone (arrow). Lower: Brain window setting showing ring-enhancing left frontal abscess, oedema and mass effect. Courtesy of Dr P Van Tassel.

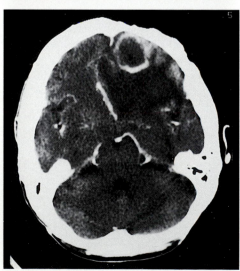

Treatment of Brain Abscess

There are relatively few direct measurements of the penetration of antimicrobial agents into brain tissue or the interior of abscess cavities; most therapeutic recommendations are based upon studies of penetration into CSF. Penicillin G in large doses (24 million units per day intravenously) is recommended because of the frequency with which streptococci are isolated from brain abscesses, even though this agent does not cross the blood–brain barrier very well. Metronidazole and chloramphenicol (active against anaerobes), third generation cephalosporins (active against many facultative Gram-negative bacilli) and trimethoprim–sulphamethoxazole (active against nocardia and many Gram-negative bacilli) are appropriate choices for combination with penicillin G in various clinical and epidemiologic settings. Amphotericin B, 5-fluorocytosine and the new triazoles, fluconazole and itraconazole, are the agents most active against fungal causes of brain abscess. In most cases drainage of the abscess should be carried out in conjunction with antimicrobial therapy. In posterior fossa lesions or fungal infections, total excision of the abscess is probably indicated. In other situations aspiration of the abscess, especially in conjunction with stereotaxic CT guidance, may be very effective. In most cases instillation of antibiotics into the abscess cavity is probably not indicated, since with a number of agents there is a risk of provoking seizures, but when highly resistant species such as *Pseudomonas aeruginosa* are implicated this may be the only way to obtain adequate local concentrations of the antimicrobial agent.

RELATED PYOGENIC INFECTIONS

Subdural Empyema

Subdural empyema is a bacterial infection in the potential space between the dura and arachnoid meninges (Fig. 7.54). It usually arises by direct extension from infection in the frontal or ethmoid sinuses, with spread from the middle ear and mastoid being less common. Streptococci and staphylococci have been isolated most frequently, but Gram-negative bacteria are found in a significant number of cases, and *Haemophilus influenzae* is relatively frequent in children under five years of age. When careful attention is paid to microbiological methods, anaerobic bacteria are often found, and polymicrobial infections are common. Most infections involve the cerebral hemispheres (see Fig. 7.54). Contiguous osteomyelitis, epidural abscess and septic venous thrombosis with haemorrhagic infarction are relatively frequent complications. The clinical picture resembles that of meningitis or brain abscess, with fever, severe headache, vomiting and

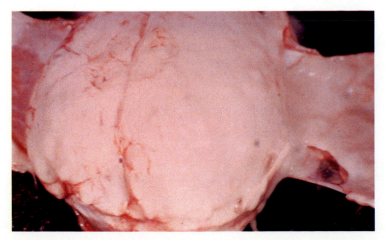

7.54 Subdural empyema. Autopsy specimen showing bilateral subdural empyemas over the cerebral hemispheres of a child.

nuchal rigidity, with rapid progression to focal neurological deficits, especially hemiparesis. Unless surgical treatment is undertaken promptly, the neurological picture progresses and herniation of the brain may occur.

Because of the rapidly increasing intracranial pressure, lumbar puncture is contraindicated. CT scanning and MRI are the most valuable diagnostic tests for this disease (Fig. 7.55); MRI is significantly more sensitive than CT scanning for the demonstration of subdural empyema. Skull films may reveal evidence of associated sinusitis or osteomyelitis. Choice of antibiotics should be based upon the principles described above for brain abscess. Mannitol or dexamethasone may be needed for treatment of cerebral oedema. Immediate surgical drainage by craniotomy or burr holes is essential to prevent the rapid progression of neurological deterioration.

Spinal subdural empyema is rare and usually arises from haematogenous spread from a focus of infection outside the nervous system. *S. aureus* is the most common aetiological agent. The clinical picture shows cord compression and/or radicular pain. MRI is the most sensitive diagnostic procedure available; myelography is the procedure of choice if MRI is not available. Therapy should consist of prompt surgical drainage and high dose treatment with a penicillinase-resistant anti-staphylococcal penicillin.

Epidural Abscess

When infection occurs between the dura and the overlying bone of the skull or vertebral column, the result is an epidural abscess (Figs 7.56 & 7.57). There is almost always associated osteomyelitis (Figs 7.58, 7.59 & 7.60), and the infection may extend through the dura into the subdural space with the formation of a concomitant subdural empyema. *S. aureus* is the infecting organism in approximately 75% of cases. The clinical picture and diagnostic and therapeutic considerations are similar to those which apply to subdural empyema.

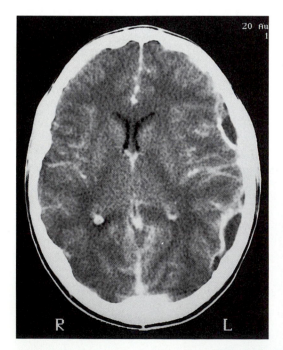 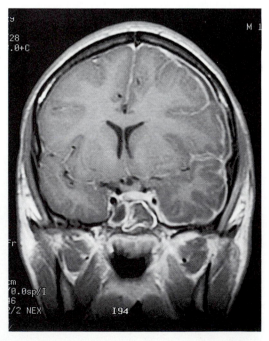

Fig. 7.55 Subdural empyema. Left: Post-contrast CT scan demonstrating abnormal rim-enhancing extra-axial fluid collections and mass effect in a patient with subdural empyemas related to acute sinusitis. Right: A post-contrast coronal MRI also shows the left-sided subdural empyemas, enhancement of the dura and the pial surface of the brain, and mass effect. Courtesy of Dr P Van Tassel.

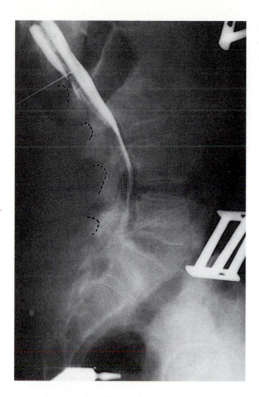

Fig. 7.56 Spinal epidural abscess. Lumbar myelogram showing anterior displacement of the column of contrast material by a posterior epidural abscess. Courtesy of Dr GD Hungerford.

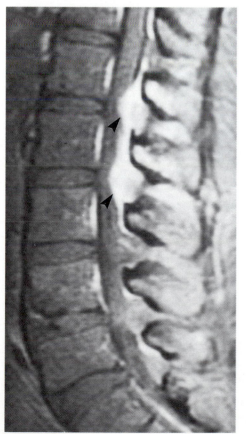

Fig. 7.57 Epidural abscess in a renal transplant patient with staphylococcal bacteraemia. This T1-weighted post-contrast sagittal MRI (with fat suppression) reveals loculated, enhancing epidural masses dorsal to the thecal sac at levels L1 to L3 (arrowheads). Courtesy of Dr P Van Tassel.

Septic Venous Thrombosis

Infection of the face, pharynx, perinasal sinuses or middle ear may spread to intracranial veins and venous sinuses by way of the emissary veins, or these structures may be involved during the course of purulent meningitis, subdural empyema or epidural abscess. The most common causative organism is *S. aureus*. The end result is venous thrombosis and suppuration, sometimes complicated by septic embolization to the lungs or other organs. Cortical vein thrombosis may produce focal neurological deficits, including hemiplegia. Cavernous sinus thrombosis produces a rapidly progressive syndrome of diplopia,

orbital oedema, exophthalmos, ophthalmoplegia and loss of vision. Thrombosis of the superior sagittal sinus results in bilateral leg weakness and can cause communicating hydrocephalus. Thrombosis of the lateral sinus produces pain over the ear and mastoid and may also result in facial pain and sixth nerve palsy. The diagnosis may be suspected when one of the syndromes described above is present in association with an extracranial focus of infection. MRI gives the most accurate visualization and localization of the thrombosed venous structures. Culture of blood and CSF may allow specific identification of the aetiological agent. Antibiotic therapy should be based upon results of culture whenever possible; if

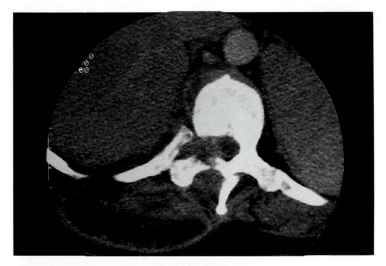

Fig. 7.58 Cryptococcosis. CT scan of vertebral body showing destructive osteomyelitis and paravertebral and epidural abscesses caused by *Cryptococcus neoformans*. Courtesy of Dr J Curé.

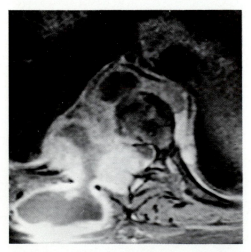

Fig. 7.59 Cryptococcosis. MRI scan of same patient showing paravertebral and epidural abscesses, destructive osteomyelitis and involvement of the spinal cord. Courtesy of Dr J Curé.

the infecting organism has not been isolated, a regimen against *S. aureus*, streptococci and anaerobic bacteria should be used. Surgical drainage and treatment of increased intracranial pressure may be required. If the disease progresses in spite of these therapeutic measures anticoagulation or surgical thrombectomy should be considered.

NEUROLOGICAL MANIFESTATIONS OF INFECTIVE ENDOCARDITIS

The friable vegetations of infective endocarditis (Fig. 7.61) may break off and produce embolic lesions in the brain, as well as in the skin and other organs (Figs 7.62, 7.63 & 7.64), and deposition of immune

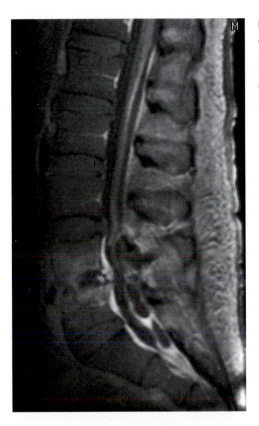

Fig. 7.60 Arachnoiditis. Diabetic patient with staphylococcal discitis, osteomyelitis and arachnoiditis. Post-contrast T1-weighted sagittal MRI (with fat suppression) showing abnormal enhancement in L4, L5 and the intervening disc space. There is also prominent epidural enhancement and abnormal clumping and enhancement of the cauda equina behind L4, L5 and S1. Courtesy of Dr P Van Tassel.

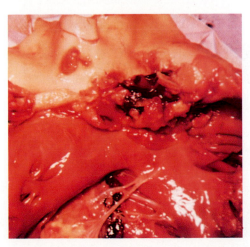

Fig. 7.61 Acute right-sided *Staphylococcus aureus* endocarditis in a 24-year-old heroin addict. Destructive vegetations can be seen on the pulmonary valve. Courtesy of Dr TF Sellers, Jr.

complexes in vessel walls may result in vascular lesions (Fig. 7.65). Neurological manifestations occur in 20–40% of patients with infective endocarditis and major neurological complications are especially common in *S. aureus* infections. Major cerebral emboli are seen in 10–30% of patients and may result in hemiplegia, aphasia, ataxia, sensory loss, alteration in mental status or a variety of neuropsychiatric manifestations. Severe headache, seizures, visual changes, movement disorders, mononeuropathy and cranial nerve palsies also occur. Mycotic aneurysms (resulting from infection of the vessel wall) are usually small, single and peripheral, and are typically silent until rupture occurs, resulting in catastrophic intracerebral or subarachnoid haemorrhage. Pathologically, embolization may result in microabscesses (Figs 7.66 & 7.67), septic infarction (Figs 7.68 & 7.69) or mycotic aneurysm. If infection spreads to the subarachnoid space to produce a meningitis, severe vasculitis may be seen (Fig. 7.70). Rupture of a mycotic aneurysm (Fig. 7.71) results in massive haemorrhage into the brain or ventricular system (Figs 7.72 & 7.73).

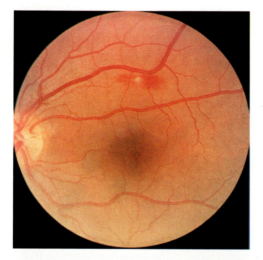

Fig. 7.62 Roth spot in bacterial endocarditis. Fundus photograph showing haemorrhage with a white centre.

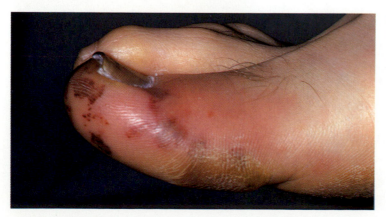

Fig. 7.63 Bacterial endocarditis. Ecchymotic embolic Janeway lesions in *Staphylococcus aureus* endocarditis. Courtesy of Dr H Tubbs.

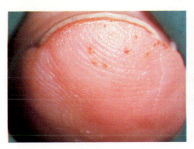
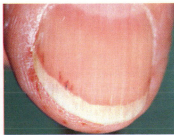

Fig. 7.64 Bacterial endocarditis. Splinter haemorrhages and petechial lesions. Courtesy of Dr H Tubbs.

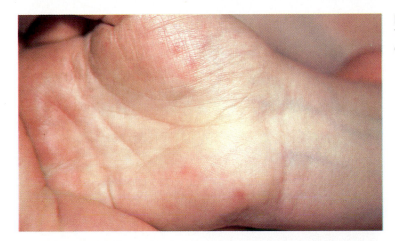

Fig. 7.65 Bacterial endocarditis. Tender Osler's nodes on the palm. Courtesy of Dr H Tubbs.

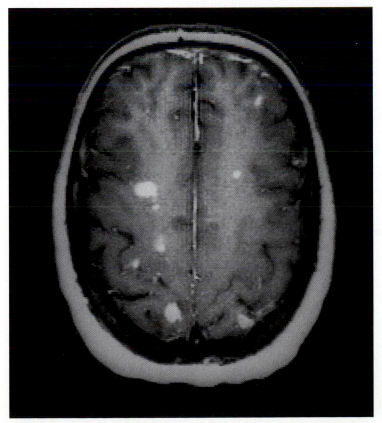

Fig. 7.66 Bacterial endocarditis. Patient with rheumatic heart disease, staphylococcal bacteraemia and septic emboli to the brain. Post-contrast T1-weighted MRI shows numerous small enhancing nodules, many of which are at corticomedullary junctions, representing abscesses. Courtesy of Dr P Van Tassel.

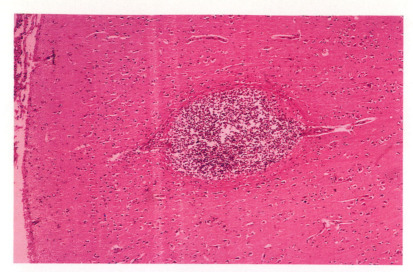

Fig. 7.67 Bacterial endocarditis. Microabscess in the cerebral cortex of a patient with endocarditis of the mitral valve due to *Staphylococcus aureus* infection. Courtesy of Dr H Okazaki and Dr B Scheithauer.

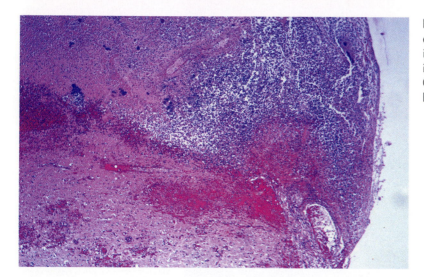

Fig. 7.68 Bacterial endocarditis. Superficial septic infarct showing intense acute inflammatory reaction. H&E stain. Courtesy of Dr H Okazaki and Dr B Scheithauer.

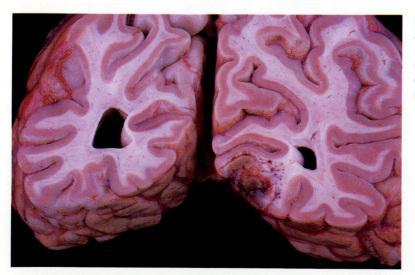

Fig. 7.69 Bacterial endocarditis. Gross specimen showing haemorrhagic infarct in the right temporal lobe. Courtesy of Dr H Okazaki and Dr B Scheithauer.

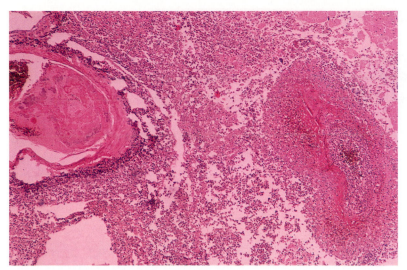

Fig. 7.70 Bacterial endocarditis. Microscopic section from the same case showing severe vasculitis in a zone of focal leptomeningitis overlying the infarct. H&E stain. Courtesy of Dr H Okazaki and Dr B Scheithauer.

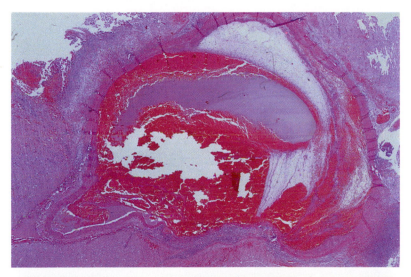

Fig. 7.71 Bacterial endocarditis. Ruptured mycotic aneurysm showing disruption of vessel wall and haemorrhage. H&E stain. Courtesy of Dr H Okazaki and Dr B Scheithauer.

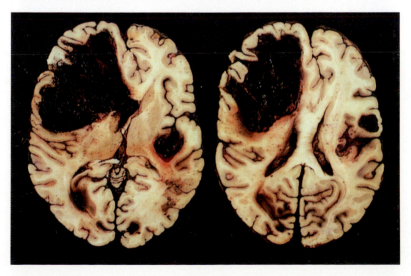

Fig. 7.72 Bacterial endocarditis. Gross specimen showing large and small haemorrhages throughout the brain, due to rupture of mycotic aneurysms. Courtesy of Dr H Okazaki and Dr B Scheithauer.

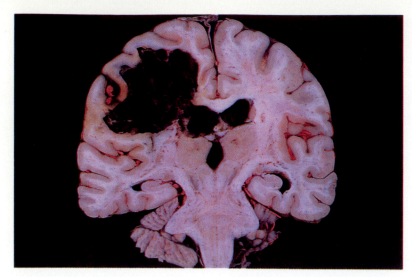

Fig. 7.73 Gross specimen from a case of ruptured mycotic aneurysm of a branch of the middle cerebral artery, with massive intracerebral haemorrhage which has ruptured into the lateral ventricle. Courtesy of Dr H Okazaki and Dr B Scheithauer.

Chapter 8

Specific Bacterial and Rickettsial Infections

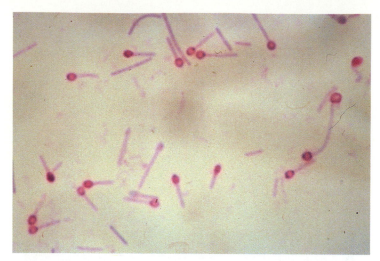

Fig. 8.1 *Clostridium tetani.* This organism is a slender bacillus which forms terminal spores, giving a 'drumstick' appearance. Spore formation occurs in tissues. Gram's stain.

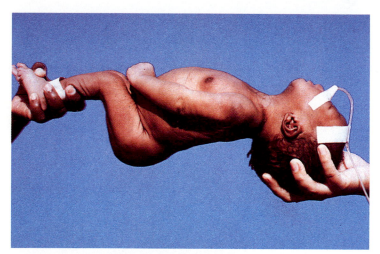

Fig. 8.2 Tetanus. Opisthotonus in an infant due to intense contraction of the paravertebral muscles. Courtesy of Dr TF Sellers, Jr.

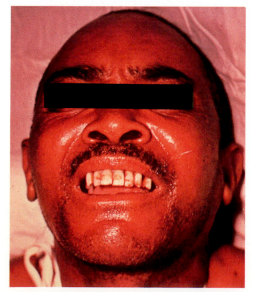

Fig. 8.3 Tetanus. Risus sardonicus, due to spasm of the facial muscles. Courtesy of Dr TF Sellers, Jr.

TETANUS

Tetanus is caused by an extremely potent neuro-toxin, tetanospasmin, produced by the anaerobic spore-forming bacterium, *Clostridium tetani*. Tetanospasmin is produced by vegetative cells of *C. tetani*, and enters the nervous system at the myoneural junctions. From there it travels centripetally along the axon to the spinal cord and then migrates transsynaptically to other neurons. Its most important action is the prevention of neurotransmitter release in synapses of inhibitory cells; this allows motor neurons to increase muscle tone unopposed and leads to muscular rigidity and spasm. Loss of inhibition within the autonomic nervous system may result in markedly elevated levels of plasma catecholamines.

C. tetani is a motile, Gram-positive, anaerobic rod. It forms terminal spores (Fig. 8.1) which are highly resistant to heat and chemical disinfectants. The organism is a normal inhabitant of the gastrointestinal tract in humans and many other mammals, and the spores may remain viable for many years in soil that has been contaminated with faeces. When spores of *C. tetani* enter the body via trauma, whether or not tetanus develops depends primarily on the immunization status of the individual, and whether or not local conditions in the wound are favourable for germination of the spores and subsequent release of toxin. Wounds contaminated with dirt, faeces or saliva, puncture wounds, and wounds associated with extensive damage to tissues, especially if other facultative microorganisms are also present, are most likely to result in the development of tetanus.

The disease is most common in developing countries where the proportion of individuals who have received effective immunization is small. Most of these cases occur in children secondary to wounds or chronic ear infections, in neonates in which the umbilical stump has been contaminated, after parturition or abortion, and following various surgical procedures performed with non-sterile instruments. In industrialized countries most cases occur in unimmunized or inadequately immunized individuals over the age of 50, in association with acute or chronic wounds, skin ulcers, abscesses, gangrene or parenteral drug abuse. In a small proportion of cases no portal of entry is evident.

The incubation period (time between injury and occurrence of the first symptom) is usually less than two weeks, but may range from a few days to up to two months. An incubation period of less than a week, or occurrence of generalized spasms within 48 hours of the first symptoms, is associated with severe disease. An early and characteristic sign is trismus or 'lockjaw', caused by an increase in muscle tone and spasm in the masseter muscle. Muscular rigidity and reflex spasms increase in extent and finally become generalized to produce painful opisthotonos (Fig. 8.2), abdominal rigidity and the characteristic facial expression of 'risus sardonicus' (Figs 8.3, 8.4 & 8.5). Spasm of respiratory muscles may result in inadequate ventilation and hypoxaemia. The reflex

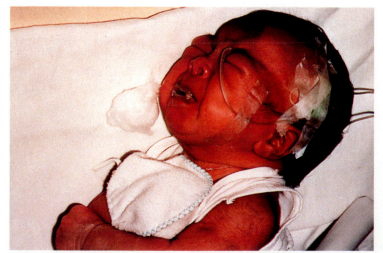

Fig. 8.4 Tetanus. Risus sardonicus in a newborn infant.

spasms may be precipitated by stimuli such as touch or changes in the level of noise or light. Autonomic dysfunction may produce labile hypertension, tachycardia, arrhythmias, profuse sweating, fever, and eventually hypotension. In uncommon cases of local tetanus the rigidity and spasms may be limited to a single extremity or to the head.

The diagnosis of tetanus depends primarily upon the characteristic clinical signs of muscle spasm and rigidity and to a lesser extent upon the history and presence of a wound. Increased tone and rigidity of the paraspinal muscles is a very helpful sign. In most cases, *C. tetani* is not isolated from cultures of the wound, and conversely the organism is sometimes isolated from wounds in patients who do not have tetanus.

Optimal treatment of tetanus requires meticulous attention to a number of important factors. Stimulation of the patient should be kept to a minimum. The constant hum of an electric fan may reduce sudden changes in the noise level, and lighting in the room should be maintained at a low but adequate level so that it is not be necessary to switch lights on and off. Benzodiazepines such as diazepam are extremely effective in inducing muscle relaxation and anxiety, and producing sedation. They should be given intravenously in small frequent doses titrated to the patient's responses. In very severe cases it may be necessary to induce neuromuscular blockade using an agent such as pancuronium bromide, but this measure greatly complicates the maintenance of respiration and handling of

secretions. If ventilatory assistance and frequent tracheal suctioning are required, tracheostomy should be performed, since this reduces the stimulation associated with these procedures. Tetanus-immune globulin (TIG) should be administered immediately (500 units intramuscularly) to neutralize any toxin which has not already entered the nervous system. Injected intrathecally, TIG (250 units) has been reported to be even more effective than when given intramuscularly. After TIG has been given, appropriate wound debridement or excision should be carried out, and treatment with either penicillin or metronidazole should be instituted. Since the amount of toxin released during clinical tetanus is insufficient to provide effective immunity, active immunization with tetanus toxoid should be initiated during hospitalization. Severe autonomic reactions may require use of adrenergic blocking agents or morphine.

There is essentially no natural immunity to tetanus, but the disease is entirely preventable by adequate immunization. Primary immunization consists of a series of injections of tetanus toxoid, either as a single agent or combined with full-dose diphtheria toxoid and/or pertussis vaccine in children, or with reduced dose diphtheria toxoid in adults. A booster injection every ten years will ensure maintenance of a protective level of antitoxin.

Appropriate prophylaxis against tetanus following a wound depends upon the individual's immune status and the nature of the wound. If the individual has both an adequate primary immunization, and

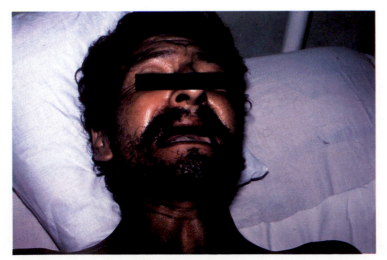

Fig. 8.5 Tetanus. Risus sardonicus in an adult.

has had a booster injection less than five years previously, no immunoprophylaxis is indicated for any type of wound. (A booster should be given if the primary immunization series used fluid toxoid.) In an immunized patient whose last booster injection was received five-to-ten years previously, no immunoprophylaxis need be given if the wound is clean, but those with a tetanus-prone wound should receive a booster. Immunized patients whose last booster injection was more than ten years previously should be given a booster with any type of wound. Individuals who have not been previously immunized should receive human TIG (250–500 units) depending on the nature and severity of the wound, and active immunization should be initiated.

BOTULISM

Botulism is a life-threatening disease, characterized by descending flaccid paralysis, caused by toxins produced by the Gram-positive, anaerobic spore-forming bacterium, *Clostridium botulinum*. These toxins, of which there are eight distinct types, are the most potent toxins known. All are polypeptides with a molecular mass of approximately 150 000 Daltons. Types A, B and E are the most common causes of botulism in man. Botulism occurs in three forms:

- Food poisoning, which results from eating food that contains the toxin.
- Wound botulism, which occurs when toxin is produced by organisms contaminating a wound.
- Infant botulism, due to toxin production by organisms within the gastrointestinal tract of infants.

Botulism food poisoning was formerly associated primarily with ingestion of sausage, but at the present time more cases are related to home-canned foods. Type E botulism is usually associated with fish products such as gefilte fish. These toxins interfere with neurotransmission at peripheral cholinergic synapses by binding tightly to the presynaptic membrane and preventing the release of acetylcholine.

The main clinical manifestation of botulism is a symmetrical, descending flaccid paralysis which begins within hours or days of ingestion of food containing the toxin. Commonly associated findings which should strengthen the suspicion of botulism are postural hypotension, dilated unreactive pupils (Fig. 8.6), ophthalmoplegia, dry mucous membranes (Fig. 8.7), and an absence of fever.

The diagnosis must be suspected on clinical grounds, and special studies are required to confirm it. Electromyography may reveal suggestive features such as decreased amplitude of the evoked muscle action potential to a single supramaximal nerve stimulus, as well as enhanced post-tetanic facilitation, muscle fibrillation, and small-amplitude polyphasic motor unit potentials of increased number and brief duration. The diagnosis may be confirmed by demonstration of toxin in the blood, toxin and/or *C. botulinum* organisms in stool or gastric contents, or toxin and/or organisms in the suspect food item. Toxin is detected by bioassay in mice. Special anaerobic culture techniques are required to isolate *C. botulinum*. Treatment consists of maintenance of airway and ventilation, general supportive care and administration of specific antitoxin. When the toxin type is unknown a trivalent ABE antitoxin should be

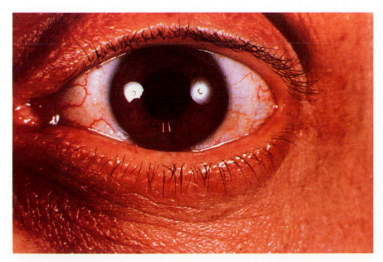

Fig. 8.6 Botulism. The characteristic dilated fixed pupil. Courtesy of Dr Z McGee.

used (available in the USA from the Centers for Disease Control, and in the UK from the Central Public Health Laboratory at Colindale). Guanidine hydrochloride has appeared to produce clinical benefit in approximately half the patients who have received it.

Wound botulism is a rare condition in which botulinum toxin is produced by organisms within a wound. The clinical picture resembles that of botulism food poisoning. Toxin may be demonstrated in the serum and occasionally *C. botulinum* can be isolated from the wound. Treatment consists of the measures described above plus surgical debridement or excision of the wound.

Infant botulism, now recognized as the most common form of botulism in the USA, is due to the release of toxin by microorganisms present within the infant's gut. The clinical picture includes constipation, generalized hypotonia, a weak and altered cry, muscle weakness, and areflexia. Ingestion of honey containing spores of *C. botulinum* appears to be a common source of infection. Treatment consists of support of respiration; most infants recover without treatment with antitoxin.

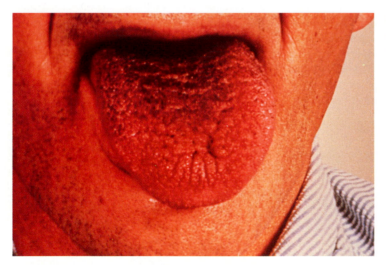

Fig. 8.7 Botulism. Clinical photograph showing dry furrowed tongue. Courtesy of Dr Z McGee.

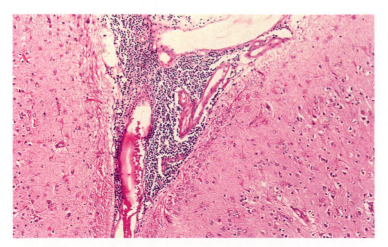

Fig. 8.8 Neurosyphilis. Meningovascular involvement in tertiary syphilis demonstrating lymphoplasmacytic meningeal infiltrate in sulcus. There is neuronal loss and marked gliosis in the underlying cortex. H&E stain. Courtesy of Dr P Garen.

NEUROSYPHILIS

During its early stages, syphilis invades the CNS in up to 40% of patients. A significant proportion of these develop persistent active infection of the CNS (neurosyphilis). Patients with asymptomatic neurosyphilis have no clinical manifestations of the disease, but do have one or more abnormalities in the CSF, including pleocytosis, elevated protein concentration, decreased glucose concentration or a positive VDRL test. Symptomatic neurosyphilis includes meningovascular and parenchymatous forms. Meningovascular syphilis is characterized by an obliterative endarteritis affecting the small blood vessels of the meninges, brain and spinal cord (Figs 8.8, 8.9, 8.10 & 8.11) resulting in multiple small areas of

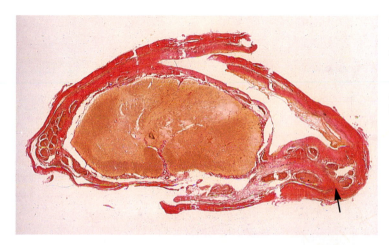

Fig. 8.9 Syphilitic pachymeningitis. Section showing cervical cord with collagenous thickening of dura and leptomeninges, particularly around the nerve roots (arrowed). Haematoxylin and Van Gieson stain. × 4. Courtesy of Dr GD Perkin.

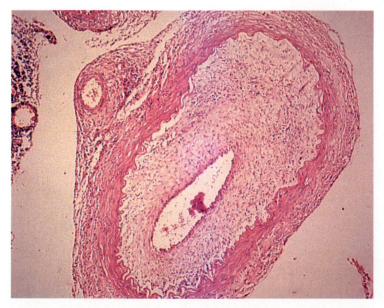

Fig. 8.10 Meningovascular syphilis. Cerebral artery showing intimal hyperplasia. H&E stain. × 60. Courtesy of Dr GD Perkin.

infarction. The most common clinical manifestations are focal neurological deficits including hemiparesis and aphasia, and focal or generalized seizures. Parenchymatous neurosyphilis includes general paresis and tabes dorsalis. In general paresis there is invasion of the brain substance by spirochaetes with destruction of nerve cells, principally in the cerebral cortex (Figs 8.12, 8.13 & 8.14). Common manifestations are changes in personality, intellect, affect and judgment, with hyperactive

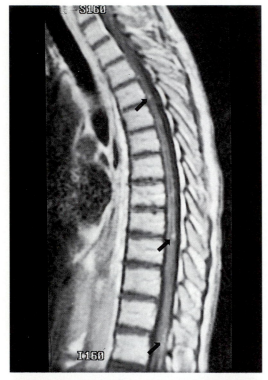

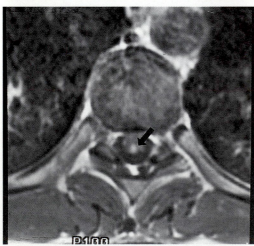

Fig. 8.11 Neurosyphilis. Post-contrast sagittal (upper) and axial (lower) T1-weighted MRI in a patient with syphylitic meningomyelitis. Note the small superficial enhancing nodules (arrows).

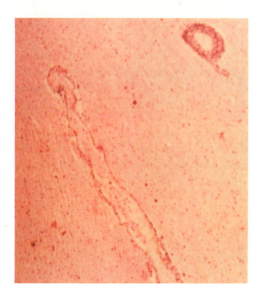

Fig. 8.12 Parenchymatous syphilis. Primarily degenerative lesion within the cerebral cortex. H&E stain.

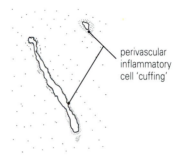

perivascular inflammatory cell 'cuffing'

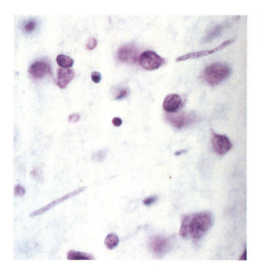

Fig. 8.13 General paresis. Histological section of the frontal cortex revealing elongate nuclei of microglial rod cells. Nissl stain.

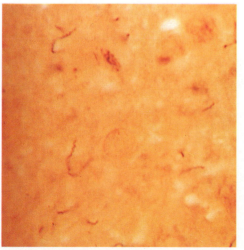

Fig. 8.14 General paresis. Histological section of the frontal cortex showing the 'corkscrew' appearance of spirochaetes. Levaditi silver stain.

reflexes, Argyll Robertson pupil and optic atrophy (Fig. 8.15). Tabes dorsalis is characterized by demyelination of the posterior column of the spinal cord, dorsal root ganglia and dorsal roots (Fig. 8.16), resulting in eventual development of a broad-based ataxic gait, foot slap, paraesthesias, lightning pains, positive Romberg's sign, hyporeflexia, degenerative joint disease (Charcot's joint), impotence, disturbance of bowel and bladder function and sensory losses. Other forms of syphilitic involvement of the central nervous system include: localized gummas of the brain or spinal cord (Fig. 8.17); syphilitic otitis, with sensorineural hearing loss or vestibular dysfunction; and syphilitic disease of the eye, pre-

senting as uveitis, chorioretinitis or episcleritis. Asymptomatic or symptomatic neurosyphilis is a relatively common late manifestation of congenital syphilis. Definitive aetiological diagnosis of syphilitic infection of the nervous system depends upon serological studies. A positive VDRL test in the CSF indicates active neurosyphilis. A titre of specific anti-treponemal IgG antibody in the spinal fluid which is at least three times higher than that in the serum, with correction for leakage of serum proteins across the blood–brain barrier, also provides strong evidence of active infection in the CNS.

Every patient with syphilis should have an examination of the CSF. If there are any abnormalities

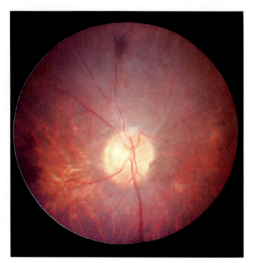

Fig. 8.15 Neurosyphilis. Fundus photograph showing optic atrophy. Courtesy of Dr MJ Wood.

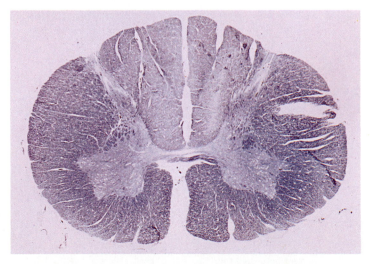

Fig. 8.16 Neurosyphilis. Degeneration of posterior columns of spinal cord in tabes dorsalis. Myelin stain. Courtesy of Dr H Whitwell.

then the patient should be treated for neurosyphilis, even if there are no clinical signs of the disease. Recommended treatment is high-dose penicillin G given intravenously for ten days. Acceptable alternative agents are ceftriaxone, doxycycline, or the combination of oral amoxicillin and probenecid. Patients with HIV infection, including those who have not progressed to AIDS, are significantly more susceptible to infection of the nervous system by *Treponema pallidum*. Many authorities therefore recommend that all patients infected with both HIV and *T. pallidum* receive treatment for neurosyphilis, preferably with a bactericidal agent such as penicillin G or ceftriaxone.

LYME DISEASE

Neurological abnormalities may be prominent in Lyme disease. The causative organism, *Borrelia burgdorferi*, like the spirochaetes of syphilis and leptospirosis, frequently reaches the CSF and tissues of the CNS early in the course of the infection. The microbiological diagnosis of neuroborreliosis is made by finding a high titre of antibody against *B. burgdorferi*, or by demonstrating *B. burgdorferi*-specific oligoclonal bands, in the CSF. Early in the infection there is often a flu-like syndrome with fever, headache, myalgias and stiff neck. The skin lesions of erythema chronicum migrans (Figs 8.18 & 8.19)

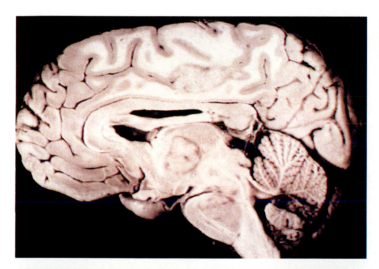

Fig. 8.17 Gumma of brain. Well-circumscribed solid mass in the thalamus of a patient with tertiary syphilis.

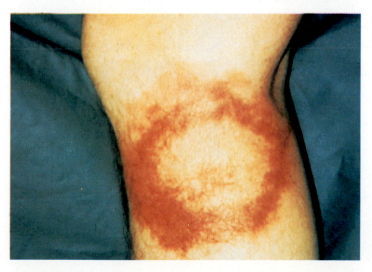

Fig. 8.18 Lyme disease. Rash of erythema chronicum migrans on leg. Courtesy of Dr E Sahn.

are characteristic, but may be absent. At this stage the CSF findings are usually normal. Later a lymphocytic meningitis with involvement of various cranial nerves (especially Bell's palsy) and a radiculoneuritis may occur. These manifestations usually respond to antibiotic therapy. Ceftriaxone appears to be more effective than penicillins or tetracyclines. Months or years later the patient may develop a chronic progressive encephalomyelitis, distal paraesthesias or radicular pain. Serious late neurological abnormalities appear to be more common in Europe than in the USA. When treating these late complications of Lyme disease, ceftriaxone, continued for at least two weeks, appears to be more effective than penicillins or other agents. Antimicrobial therapy is clearly more effective if given early in the course of the disease.

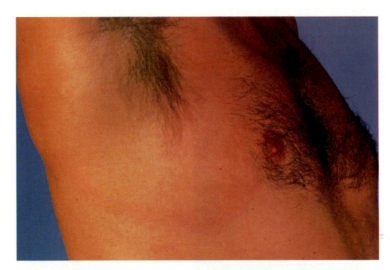

Fig. 8.19 Lyme disease. Margin of large erythema chronicum migrans lesion extending over chest wall and around axilla. Courtesy of Dr VE del Bene.

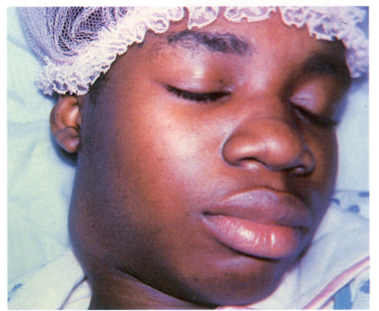

Fig. 8.20 Cat scratch disease. Large cervical lymph nodes in a drowsy patient with complicating encephalitis. Courtesy of Dr TF Sellers, Jr.

CAT SCRATCH DISEASE

Encephalopathy occurs in approximately 1% of patients with cat scratch disease (Fig. 8.20). Seizures (50%), combative behaviour (40%), lethargy (rarely progressing to coma) and headache are common manifestations. Mild pleocytosis and increased protein concentration in the CSF are each seen in about a third of cases. CT scan is usually normal, but discrete lesions have been seen on MRI scan (Fig. 8.21), and diffuse slowing is observed on EEG in 80%. Cranial neuropathies, including Bell's palsy and neuroretinitis, and peripheral neuritis occur only rarely.

Most, if not all, cases of cat scratch disease appear to be due to the rickettsia-like organism *Rochalimaea henselae*, but the bacterium, *Afipia felis*, may cause a minority of cases. Bacillary organisms may sometimes be seen in tissues, especially lymph nodes, using Warthin–Starry stain (Fig. 8.22).

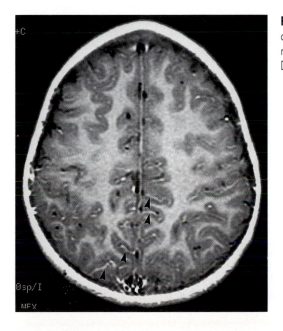

Fig. 8.21 Cat scratch disease. T1-weighted post-contrast MRI in a child with clinical evidence of cat scratch disease and seizures, revealing subtle meningeal enhancement (arrowheads). Courtesy of Dr P Van Tassel.

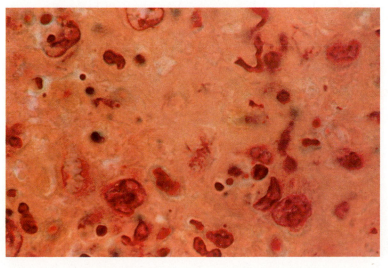

Fig. 8.22 Cat scratch disease. Bacilli in a lymph node. Warthin–Starry stain.

LEPROSY

Peripheral nerve involvement in leprosy is manifested by thickened superficial nerves (Fig. 8.23) and, especially in tuberculoid leprosy, anaesthesia of the cutaneous lesions (Fig. 8.24) The anaesthesia may lead to ulceration and loss of tissue (Fig. 8.25) . In tuberculoid leprosy the nerve bundles are infiltrated with mononuclear inflammatory cells but few bacilli are present (Fig. 8.26) . In the lepromatous form acid-fast bacilli are abundant (Fig. 8.27).

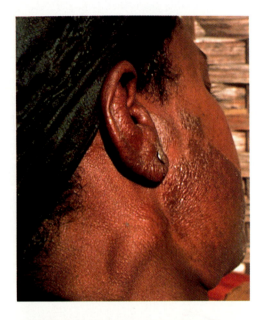

Fig. 8.23 Leprosy. Enlargement of the great auricular nerve in relationship to inflamed borderline tuberculoid lesions.

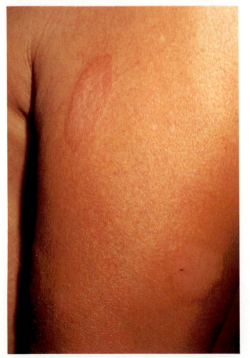

Fig. 8.24 Leprosy. Skin lesions of borderline tuberculoid (BT) leprosy showing a raised erythematous margin. The centre of the lesion was anaesthetic. A similar solitary lesion is typical of tuberculoid (TT) disease. Courtesy of Dr CJ Ellis.

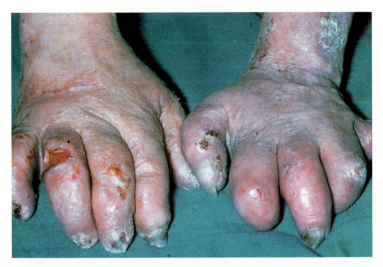

Fig. 8.25 Leprosy. Hands in advanced untreated leprosy showing gross deformity and loss of tissue.

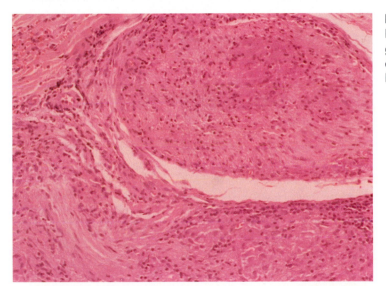

Fig. 8.26 Tuberculoid leprosy. Peripheral nerve expanded by granulomatous inflammation. Giant cells are present in the nerve bundle. H&E stain. Courtesy of Dr P Garen.

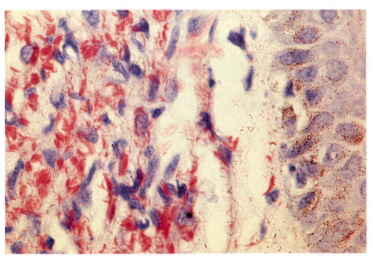

Fig. 8.27 Lepromatous leprosy. Histology of skin biopsy showing clumps of acid-fast bacilli (stained red) in the dermis. Ziehl–Neelsen stain. Courtesy of Dr CJ Ellis.

ROCKY MOUNTAIN SPOTTED FEVER

Significant neurological involvement is common in Rocky Mountain spotted fever. Most patients complain of severe headache and photophobia; focal neurological deficits, transient deafness, stiff neck, stupor, and papilloedema without increased CSF pressure, are also seen. CSF pleocytosis (usually lymphocytic) and increased protein concentration occur in approximately a third of patients. EEG may show evidence of diffuse cortical dysfunction. Prominent neurological involvement is associated with an increased case-fatality rate and a high incidence of residual neurological sequelae, especially if appropriate antimicrobial therapy is not started promptly. In 10–15% of patients the characteristic rash (Figs 8.28 & 8.29) either develops late in the course of the illness or is absent, making it extremely difficult to

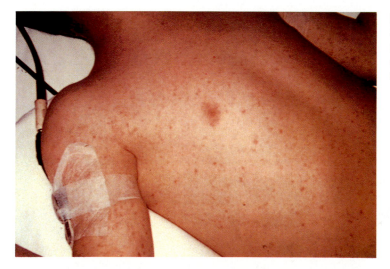

Fig. 8.28 Rocky Mountain spotted fever. Seventh day of illness in a small boy. A moderately severe eruption with macular and petechial elements of various size. Courtesy of Dr TF Sellers, Jr.

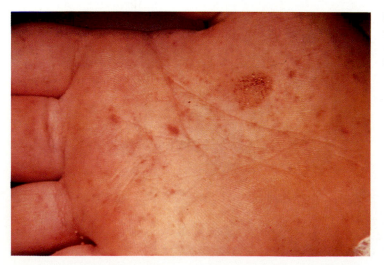

Fig. 8.29 Rocky Mountain spotted fever. Hand of patient shown in Fig. 8.28, on the seventh day of illness. Courtesy of Dr TF Sellers, Jr.

distinguish this disease from other forms of encephalitis. The characteristic lesion is a vasculitis and perivasculitis due to direct invasion of vascular endothelial cells by the rickettsiae (Fig. 8.30), with secondary microinfarction of brain tissue (Fig. 8.31). Encephalitis has also been seen in cases of *Rickettsia conorii* infection (*fièvre boutonneuse*).

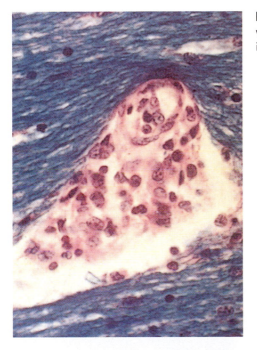

Fig. 8.30 Rocky Mountain spotted fever. Vasculitis in a small blood vessel with prominent perivascular clustering of mononuclear inflammatory cells to form a 'typhus nodule'. Luxol-fast blue, H&E stain.

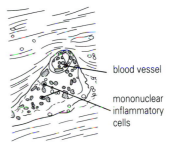

Fig. 8.31 Rocky Mountain spotted fever. Microinfarct in the white matter of the brain of a child. The small infarcts are caused by the vasculitis characteristic of this disease. Luxol-fast blue, H&E stain.

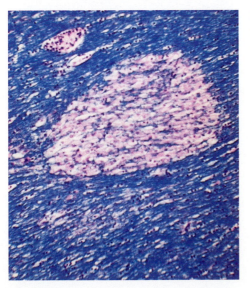

Chapter 9

Specific Parasitic Infections

TOXOPLASMOSIS

The protozoan parasite *Toxoplasma gondii* is a common cause of latent infection of the central nervous system throughout the world. Domestic cats and other felines are the definitive hosts, but humans (and many other mammals) acquire the infection incidentally by ingestion of oocysts in cat faeces, ingestion of tissue cysts in infected meat or by transmission *in utero*. Clinically apparent infection of the nervous system is seen almost exclusively in immunocompromised individuals. Although some cases of toxoplasma encephalitis have occurred in patients receiving immunosuppressing drugs, especially recipients of transplants of heart or bone marrow, this disease is the most important opportunistic CNS infection in patients with AIDS. In Western Europe about 25% of patients with AIDS develop toxoplasma encephalitis, and in many developing countries the incidence is even higher. In industrialized countries most cases occur in patients already diagnosed as having AIDS, and represent recrudescence of latent CNS infection. In developing countries with a high prevalence of toxoplasmosis,

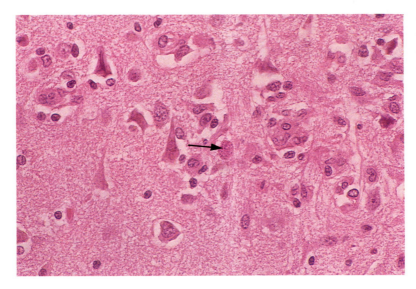

Fig. 9.1 Cerebral toxoplasmosis. Microscopic granuloma in the cerebral cortex. A single cyst containing many organisms (arrow) can be seen at the edge of the lesion. H&E stain. Courtesy of Dr H Okazaki and Dr B Scheithauer.

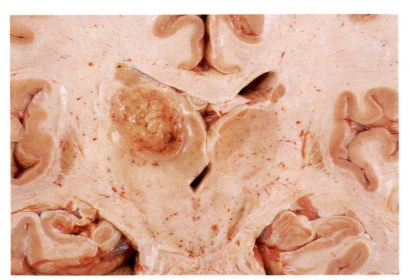

Fig. 9.2 Cerebral toxoplasmosis. Gross specimen showing a large necrotic lesion completely surrounded by a haemorrhagic border in the left thalamus. Courtesy of Dr H Okazaki and Dr B Scheithauer.

encephalitis may develop early in the course of HIV infection and may represent a recently acquired infection.

Toxoplasma encephalitis consists of multiple focal mass lesions, which may be granulomatous or necrotizing in nature, occurring in any part of the CNS but most commonly in the basal ganglia or corticomedullary junction of the cerebrum. Clinically, patients usually present with altered mental status, which may progress to coma, headache and focal neurological deficits. Seizures occur in approximately a third of patients. A syndrome of inappropriate secretion of antidiuretic hormone may be present. Examination of the CSF may reveal no abnormalities or there may be a mononuclear pleocytosis with increased protein and normal glucose.

Definitive aetiological diagnosis of toxoplasma encephalitis usually requires brain biopsy. Histopathological examination may reveal a granulomatous reaction (Fig. 9.1), or severe, necrotizing, focal or diffuse encephalitis (Figs 9.2 & 9.3). Tachyzoites (Fig. 9.4) or bradycysts (Fig. 9.5) may be seen in brain sections stained with haematoxylin and eosin, in touch preparations stained with Wright–Giemsa stain, or by specific immunohistological staining by the immunoperoxidase method

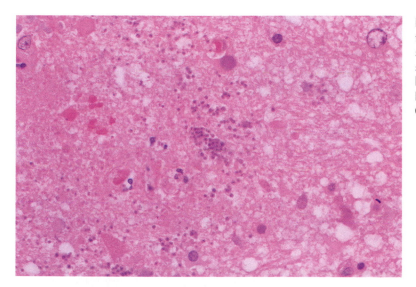

Fig. 9.3 Cerebral toxoplasmosis. Microscopic section from the same lesion, showing multiple organisms, both encysted and free. H&E stain. Courtesy of Dr H Okazaki and Dr B Scheithauer.

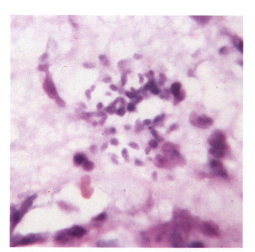

Fig. 9.4 Toxoplasma encephalitis. Histological section of brain biopsy showing numerous tachyzoites of *Toxoplasma gondii*, necrosis and inflammatory reaction. Giemsa stain. Courtesy of Dr MJ Wood.

(Fig. 9.6) – this is the most sensitive technique. Isolation of *T. gondii* from other tissue specimens or body fluids outside the CNS indicates active infection, and provides supportive evidence for the diagnosis. Approximately 97% of patients with AIDS who have toxoplasma encephalitis are seropositive when first seen, so a negative IgG antibody test in serum virtually rules out this diagnosis. An IgG antibody titre in CSF which exceeds that in the serum indicates the local production of antibody in the CNS and also strongly suggests the diagnosis of toxoplasma encephalitis. *T. gondii* can now be grown *in vitro* in tissue culture, and methods for detection of antigen in serum and CSF are being developed.

Imaging studies of the brain, especially CT scanning and MRI, may provide strong presumptive evidence of toxoplasma encephalitis. The typical finding on CT scanning is of multiple, bilateral, hypodense, enhancing mass lesions, especially in the basal ganglia and at the corticomedullary junctions of the cerebrum (Fig. 9.7). Single lesions are occasionally seen (Fig. 9.8). 'Double-dose' enhanced CT scanning may provide increased sensitivity. MRI appears to be even more sensitive than CT scanning,

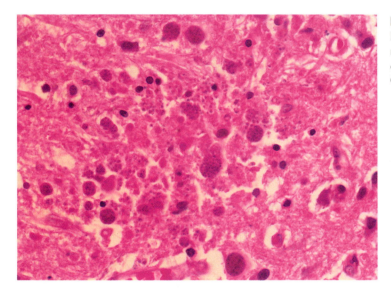

Fig. 9.5 Cerebral toxoplasmosis. Focal area of acute necrosis with numerous bradycysts and tachyzoites of *Toxoplasma gondii*. H&E stain. Courtesy of Dr P Garen.

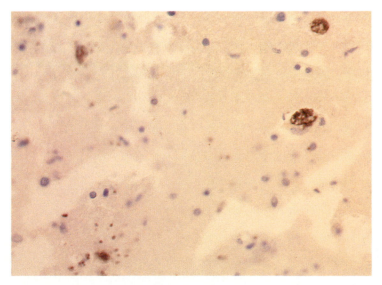

Fig. 9.6 Cerebral toxoplasmosis. Immunostaining reveals tachyzoites and bradycysts. Courtesy of Dr P Garen.

and nearly always reveals multiple lesions (Fig. 9.9). The finding of a single lesion on MRI suggests another diagnosis, such as intracerebral lymphoma.

Toxoplasma encephalitis in AIDS patients is invariably fatal if untreated, so patients with multiple focal lesions on imaging studies should receive immediate empirical treatment while additional diagnostic studies are done. Standard therapy consists of pyrimethamine plus sulfadiazine, with folinic acid to reduce the toxicity of pyrimethamine to the bone marrow. Up to 40% of patients on this regimen develop leucopenia or rash, in which case the therapy is often discontinued. Many of the adverse effects are due to the sulfadiazine; pyrimethamine plus clindamycin may be used as an alternative regimen. Patients usually show clinical improvement within two weeks, and improvement in the appearance of the imaging studies in three-to-four weeks. The primary course of therapy should be continued for at least six weeks. Since these agents do not eradicate toxoplasma cysts, the patient remains susceptible to relapse of the infection for life, and should receive suppressive treatment with either pyrimethamine/sulfadiazine or clindamycin indefinitely.

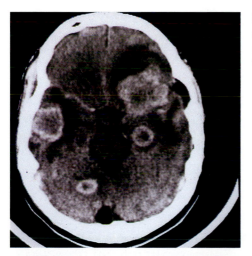

Fig. 9.7 Cerebral toxoplasmosis. CT scan showing multiple ring-enhancing, hypodense lesions in the left fronto-temporal, right temporal, right occipital and left uncal regions, with surrounding cerebral oedema. Courtesy of Dr MJ Wood.

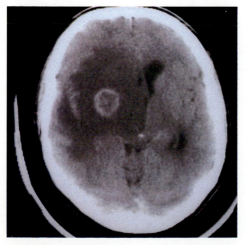

Fig. 9.8 Cerebral toxoplasmosis. CT scan showing a single ring-enhancing, hypodense lesion deep in the basal ganglia, surrounded by an extensive area of oedema. Courtesy of Dr MJ Wood.

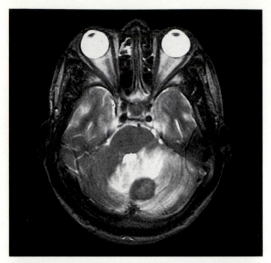

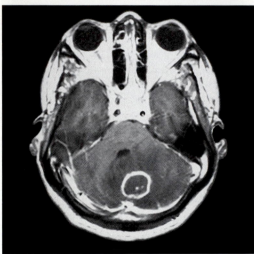

Fig. 9.9 Cerebral toxoplasmosis. Two MRIs from a patient with AIDS, demonstrating multiple intracranial lesions. Upper: T2-weighted axial image showing a hypointense mass with surrounding oedema. Lower: Post-contrast T1-weighted image demonstrating the typical ring enhancement of the lesion. These lesions improved after antibiotic therapy. Courtesy of Dr P Van Tassel.

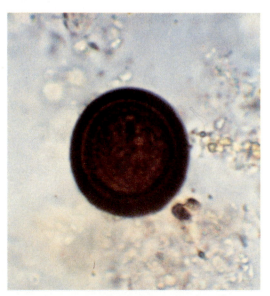

Fig. 9.10 Taeniasis. An egg of either *Taenia solium* or *Taenia saginata* in faeces containing hexacanth larvae. Courtesy of Dr TW Holbrook.

CYSTICERCOSIS

Cysticercus cellulosae is the name given to the intermediate stage of the pork tapeworm, *Taenia solium* (Fig. 9.10). Humans may become intermediate hosts for the organism by ingestion of food or water contaminated with human faeces, by self-infection from anus to mouth in a person infected with the adult tapeworm, or by internal infection due to reverse peristalsis. The oncosphere penetrates the intestinal wall and rapidly develops into a fluid-filled cyst which contains the invaginated head of the larva (Figs 9.11 & 9.12). The organism lives for several years and then dies and degenerates, after which it

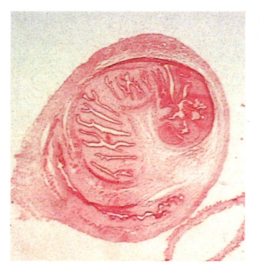

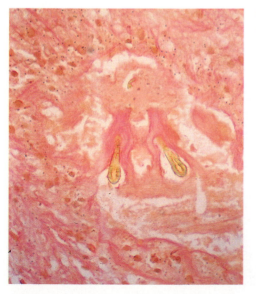

Fig. 9.11 Taeniasis. Scolex of immature *Taenia solium* in cystic lesion of cysticercosis. H&E stain.

Fig. 9.12 Cysticercosis. High power histology showing hooklets. Courtesy of Dr H Whitwell.

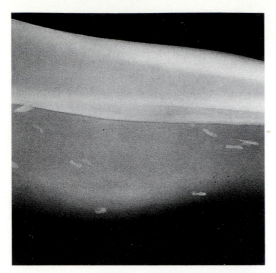

Fig. 9.13 Taeniasis. Radiograph of leg showing characteristic elongated calcified cysts of *Taenia solium*. At this site they produce no symptoms.

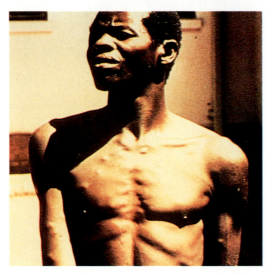

Fig. 9.14 Taeniasis. Infection with the larval form of *Taenia solium* (cysticercosis) showing multiple subcutaneous cystic lesions containing the larvae, which are known as *Cysticercus cellulosae*. Courtesy of Dr GM Schultz.

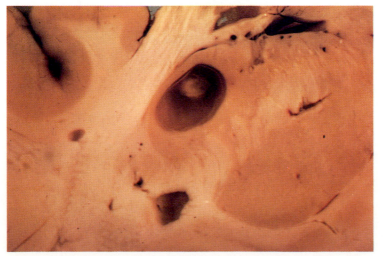

Fig. 9.15 Cerebral cysticercosis. Gross specimen of brain showing a simple cyst in the caudate nucleus. Within it can be seen the scolex of the developing tapeworm. Courtesy of Professor H Spencer.

may eventually calcify (Figs 9.13 & 9.14). The CNS is the most common clinically significant site of infection. Lesions may be focal and discrete when the cysts occur in the brain substance (Figs 9.15 & 9.16). If the infection occurs in the subarachnoid space at the base of the brain or in the ventricles, involvement is more diffuse, and this so-called racemose form may invade the surrounding tissue (Fig. 9.17). Clinically, patients may present with headache, papilloedema, decreased vision, and focal neurological signs including hemiparesis and seizures. The most useful diagnostic tests are CT scanning (Figs 9.18 & 9.19) and MRI (Figs 9.20 & 9.21), which reveal the multiple space-occupying cystic lesions and hydrocephalus. Serological tests on serum and spinal fluid are usually positive and confirm the aetiological diagnosis. Recently, praziquantel has proved effective in killing the larval stage of the organism. Patients who have active infection with living organisms usually exhibit marked and rapid improvement with treatment. If the organisms are already dead, treatment does not influence the clinical manifestations. Concurrent treatment with corticosteroids may also be beneficial.

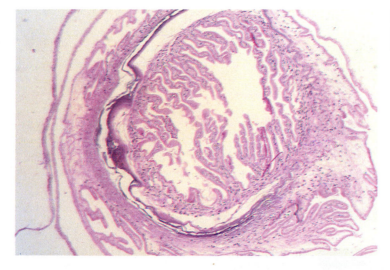

Fig. 9.16 Cysticercosis. Scolex present in lesion of brain. H&E stain. Courtesy of Dr P Garen.

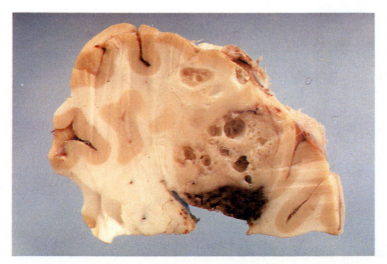

Fig. 9.17 Cerebral cysticercosis. Post-mortem specimen of brain showing racemose form with diffuse involvement of surrounding tissues. Courtesy of Professor H Spencer.

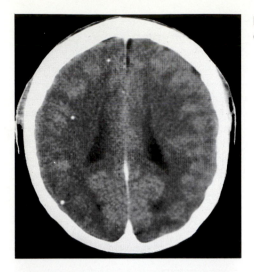

Fig. 9.18 Cerebral cysticercosis. CT scan showing three small round calcified lesions in the right cerebral hemisphere. Courtesy of Dr J Curé.

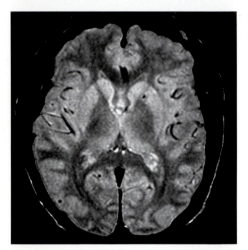

Fig. 9.19 Cerebral cysticercosis. MRI scan of same patient showing multiple small round lesions in the brain. Courtesy of Dr J Curé.

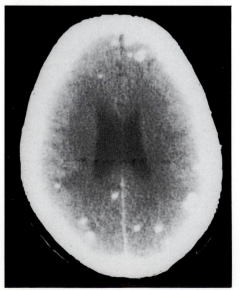

Fig. 9.20 Cerebral cysticercosis. CT scan showing multiple calcified cysts. Courtesy of Dr J Curé.

AFRICAN TRYPANOSOMIASIS

African trypanosomiasis is caused by a flagellated protozoan, *Trypanosoma brucei* (Fig. 9.22), which is transmitted from wild and domestic animals to man by tsetse flies (genus *Glossina* – Fig. 9.23). The range of the vectors (and the disease) includes the region of Africa between latitudes 15°N and 15°S. Both the West African form, caused by *T. brucei gambiense* and the East African form, caused by *T. b. rhodesiense*, cause a meningoencephalitis which is responsible for much of the morbidity and mortality associated with this disease. The West African form is usually a chronic disease lasting for many months, whereas the East African type is much more acute and stormy, with death from toxaemia occurring often within a few weeks of the onset of symptoms, before invasion of the CNS becomes apparent.

Following the bite of an infected tsetse fly, a small nodule (trypanosomal chancre) forms at the site of inoculation. Weeks or months later invasion of the bloodstream occurs with fever, general malaise, myalgia, headache, generalized lymphadenopathy (often including enlargement of the

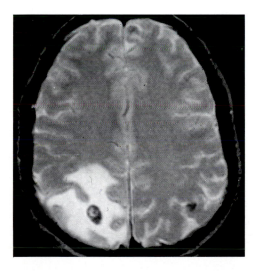

Fig. 9.21 Cerebral cysticercosis. MRI scan showing a cyst containing a developing larva, surrounded by an area of oedema. Courtesy of Dr J Curé.

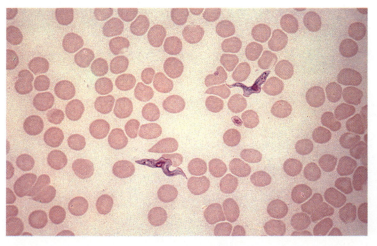

Fig. 9.22 African trypanosomiasis. Trypanosomes in a thin blood smear.

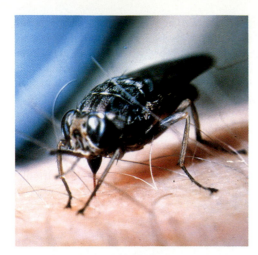

Fig. 9.23 African trypanosomiasis. Tsetse fly feeding.

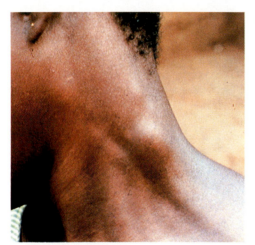

Fig. 9.24 African trypanosomiasis. Enlargement of lymph nodes in posterior cervical triangle (Winterbottom's sign). Courtesy of Professor PG Janssens.

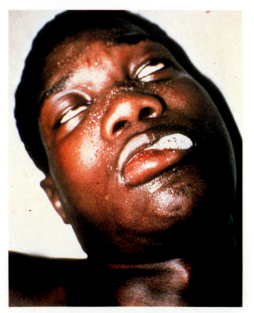

Fig. 9.25 West African sleeping sickness. Terminal coma due to generalized encephalitis. Courtesy of Dr ME Krampitz and Dr P de Raadt.

posterior cervical nodes, Winterbottom's sign, Fig. 9.24), splenomegaly, hepatomegaly and parasitaemia. During this stage of the disease (the systemic or haemolymphatic phase) the fever is usually episodic and the level of parasitaemia fluctuates. This fluctuation reflects the parasite's ability to vary its surface antigens and thus evade the host's antibody response.

The final (meningoencephalitic) stage is characterized by increasing and persistent headache, disturbance of sleep pattern, ataxia and other movement disorders, abnormal behaviour and depression of consciousness with stupor and progression to irreversible coma (Fig. 9.25). The patient eventually succumbs to an intercurrent respiratory or other infection. Pathologically, the brain reveals perivascular infiltration with mononuclear cells,

plasma cells, lymphocytes and so-called morular or Mott cells (Fig. 9.26). The Mott cell is a distinctive form of plasma cell which has large eosinophilic inclusions.

Diagnosis of African trypanosomiasis is usually made by demonstration of trypanosomes in blood during the febrile stage (see Fig. 9.22). Organisms may also be found in aspirates of lymph nodes or chancres. Serological methods of diagnosis have not proved very satisfactory, but newer tests utilizing DNA hybridization and the polymerase chain reaction are being developed. In the meningoencephalitic stage, examination of the CSF reveals a predominantly lymphocytic pleocytosis and elevated protein concentration, including elevation of IgM antibody. Mott cells and motile trypanosomes may also be found (Fig. 9.27).

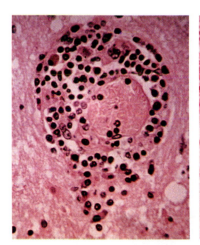
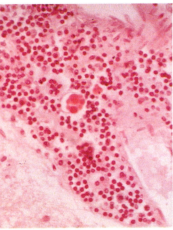

Fig. 9.26 West African sleeping sickness. Histological section of brain.
Left: Prominent perivascular infiltration ('cuffing') by mononuclear cells, lymphocytes and plasma cells. H&E stain. Courtesy of Professor MSR Hutt.
Right: A prominent Mott cell. H&E stain. Courtesy of Professor W Peters.

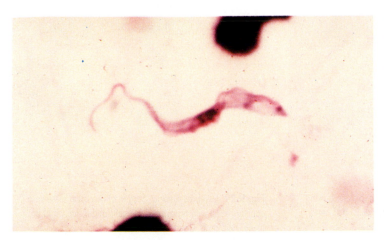

Fig. 9.27 West African sleeping sickness. Preparation of cerebrospinal fluid showing a typical trypanosome (no Mott cells are seen in this particular preparation). Giemsa stain. Courtesy of the Wellcome Museum of Medical Science.

In early stage disease, suramin is effective in eradicating infection with *T. b. rhodesiense* or *T. b. gambiense*; pentamidime is effective only in early *T. b. gambiense* infection. In late stage disease, only melarsoprol and nifurtimox have proved to be useful. All of the antitrypanosomal drugs are associated with serious toxic effects. Follow-up should be continued for at least two years to detect relapse, which is relatively common in these infections.

CEREBRAL MALARIA

Headache, irritability, confusion and (in children) febrile convulsions, occur commonly in malaria due to *Plasmodium falciparum*. However, an alteration in the level of consciousness, ranging from mild stupor to unarousable coma, may indicate the presence of a diffuse encephalopathy (cerebral malaria). Stiff neck, retinal haemorrhages, dysconjugate gaze and signs of upper motor neuron dysfunction (hypertonia, increased tendon reflexes with ankle clonus, extensor plantar response and absent abdominal reflexes) may also occur. Pathologically, there is sequestration of parasitized erythrocytes in the microvasculature of the brain (Figs 9.28 & 9.29), shown by electron microscopy to be due to cytoadherence of knob-like protuberances on the erythrocyte surface to vascular endothelium. This causes the obstruction of cerebral capillaries and venules, with the development of ring haemorrhages around some of the obstructed vessels. Decreased deformability of infected erythrocytes may also contribute to sluggish blood flow. Metabolic abnormalities, including anaerobic glycolysis in the brain and reduced cerebral oxygen transport, have also been demonstrated.

Cerebral malaria should be treated with intravenous quinine. Chloroquine, which is less toxic than quinine, may be used in areas in which only chloroquine-sensitive strains of *P. falciparum* are present. If parenteral quinine is not available then quinidine gluconate may be used; ECG and blood pressure should be monitored closely throughout the infusion period. Seizures should be managed with parenteral phenobarbital. Use of corticosteroids such as dexamethasone is contraindicated.

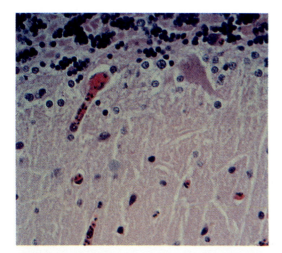

Fig. 9.28 Cerebral malaria. Section of cerebellum showing capillaries filled with parasitized red blood cells. H&E stain. Courtesy of Dr MJ Wood.

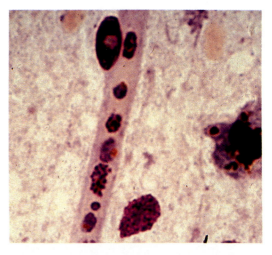

Fig. 9.29 Cerebral malaria. Section of cerebrum showing a capillary filled with parasitized red cells and infarction of brain tissue. H&E stain. Courtesy of Dr MJ Wood.

Chapter 10

Specific Viral Infections

POLIOMYELITIS

Poliomyelitis is due to infection with the polioviruses, members of the enterovirus group (Fig. 10.1). There are three serotypes of polioviruses, but it is type 1 that causes most paralytic poliomyelitis in unimmunized populations. Infection is initiated by replication of the virus in the gut and associated lymphoid tissues, followed by viraemic spread to reticuloendothelial tissues throughout the body. In most patients the infection is contained at this point and no symptoms result. In a few people replication in the reticuloendothelial system results in a major viraemia which corresponds to the non-specific febrile illness known as abortive poliomyelitis.

Viraemia may also lead to seeding of the leptomeninges, causing aseptic meningitis (non-paralytic poliomyelitis). In a small proportion of cases, spread of the virus to the nervous system may cause extensive necrosis of neurons in the grey matter of the spinal cord and brain with production of paralytic poliomyelitis. Destruction of neurons is accompanied by an inflammatory infiltrate of polymorphonuclear (PMN) leucocytes, lymphocytes and macrophages (Fig. 10.2). The major sites of attack are the anterior horn of the spinal cord and the motor nuclei of the pons and medulla.

Of all poliomyelitis infections, 99% are asymptomatic, and only 0.1% result in paralytic disease. The most common form of paralytic poliomyelitis

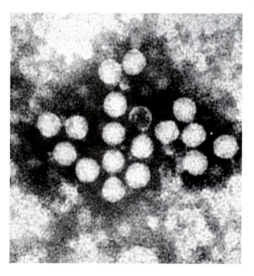

Fig. 10.1 Poliomyelitis. Electron micrograph showing spherical poliovirus particles, approximately 25 nm in diameter. Courtesy of Dr MJ Wood.

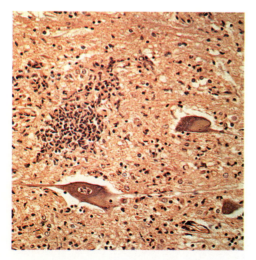

Fig. 10.2 Poliomyelitis. Histological section of spinal cord showing microglial nodules. H&E stain. Courtesy of Dr MJ Wood.

involves the spinal cord with production of an asymmetrical flaccid paralysis, which affects some muscle groups while sparing others. Proximal muscles of the extremities are most commonly involved, legs more so than arms. Bulbar poliomyelitis may involve the nuclei of cranial nerves, especially nerves IX–XII, and the respiratory and vasomotor centres. Involvement of cranial nerves may result in difficulty in swallowing and handling of secretions, and involvement of medullary centres may cause hypertension, hyperthermia, tachycardia, Cheyne–Stokes respiration and potentially fatal cardiac arrhythmias.

In developing countries in which few individuals are immunized against poliomyelitis, most cases occur in children under the age of five years. In industrialized countries, where most individuals have been immunized, infection with wild-type virus is extremely rare. Most infections are due to vaccine strains, especially types 3 and 2. Paralytic disease occurs in approximately 1 out of every 2.6 million recipients of the oral, live-virus vaccine.

Specific aetiological diagnosis of poliovirus infection can be made by isolation of the virus from throat washings in the first week of illness, or from faeces for several weeks thereafter. The organism can also be isolated from the cerebrospinal fluid (CSF), but this is rare. In the absence of virus isolation, the diagnosis can be established by demonstrating a significant rise in antibody titre during convalescence from the illness.

Since there are no specific antiviral agents which are effective in the treatment of poliovirus infections, management consists of supportive care and maintenance of adequate ventilation and an adequate airway. Both inactivated-virus vaccines and live attenuated oral vaccines are extremely effective in prevention of paralytic poliomyelitis.

GUILLAIN–BARRÉ SYNDROME

Guillain–Barré syndrome is an inflammatory demyelinating process affecting peripheral nerves, predominantly the anterior roots. It results in an ascending flaccid paralysis with paraesthesias, loss of deep tendon reflexes and muscle wasting (Fig. 10.3). Most, but not all, cases are preceded by an acute infection or immunization. A number of viruses, including influenza A virus, Epstein–Barr virus, human immunodeficiency virus (HIV) and various enteroviruses, as well as *Mycoplasma pneumoniae*, have been associated with this syndrome. The disease closely resembles experimental allergic neuritis, a disease induced in animals by immunization with peripheral nerve myelin, and may represent sensitization to this substance. A characteristic finding is an increased protein concentration in the CSF, with few or no cells (albumino-cytological dissociation). Involvement of ventilatory muscles may necessitate respiratory assistance. Involvement of the autonomic nervous system may result in labile blood pressure which is difficult to control. Many patients benefit from plasmaphaeresis, particularly if the treatment is instituted early in the disease. Improvement may occur only gradually, over a period of a year or more, but long-term prognosis is good.

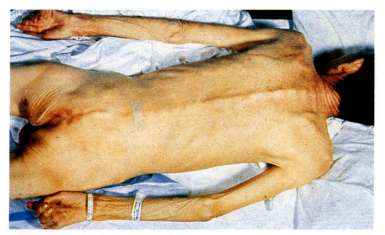

Fig. 10.3 Guillain–Barré syndrome. Limb wasting. Courtesy of Dr PO Behan.

HUMAN IMMUNODEFICIENCY VIRUS

Neurological disease occurs at some time during the course of HIV infection in nearly all individuals. Aseptic meningitis is seen in approximately 25% of cases of acute retroviral syndrome, and various cranial neuropathies without meningeal signs occur less frequently. HIV encephalopathy (Figs 10.4 & 10.5) due to involvement of the white matter of the CNS by HIV is very common, and the incidence increases with progression of HIV infection. More than 90% of patients with AIDS have cognitive, affective or psychomotor abnormalities. Early in the course of HIV encephalopathy there may be loss of memory, decreased ability to concentrate, mental slowing, affective symptoms, apathy, change in behaviour, motor complaints, increased deep tendon reflexes, hypertonia, frontal-release signs and ataxia. CT scanning reveals generalized atrophy in 70–90% of cases, and MRI is even more sensitive, revealing abnormalities in the white matter and multifocal areas of increased signal intensity (Fig. 10.6). As the disease progresses the dementia becomes more severe with marked abnormalities in cognition, profound memory loss, changes in behaviour, psychosis, weakness, tremors and, occasionally, seizures. CT scanning and MRI reveal extreme atrophy and progressive changes in the white matter. Histopathologically there is gliosis, focal necrosis, microglial nodules, demyelination and occasional multinucleated cells. Vacuolar myelopathy (Figs 10.7, 10.8 & 10.9) may occur and result in spastic paralysis of the extremities and faecal and urinary incontinence.

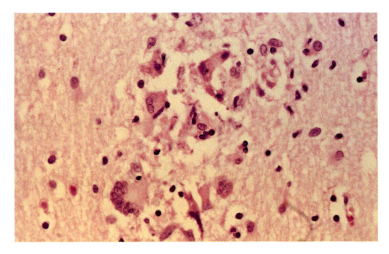

Fig. 10.4 HIV encephalopathy. Histological section of the brain showing accumulation of multinucleated giant cells in a perivascular location. H&E stain. Courtesy of Dr P Garen.

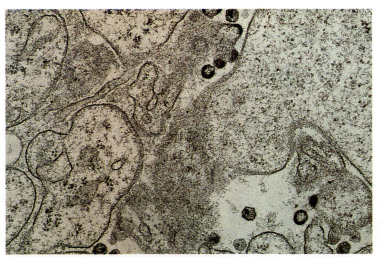

Fig. 10.5 HIV encephalopathy. Electron micrograph from stereotactic brain biopsy of a patient with AIDS dementia showing HIV viruses emerging from a multinucleated giant cell. Courtesy of Dr PO Behan.

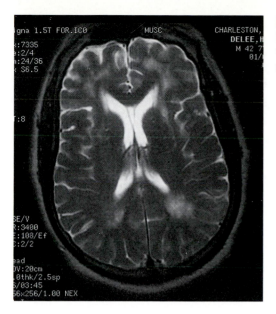

Fig. 10.6 HIV encephalopathy. T2-weighted axial MRI of the brain in an AIDS patient, showing an abnormal hyperintense signal in the white matter bilaterally, consistent with viral encephalitis. Courtesy of Dr P Van Tassl.

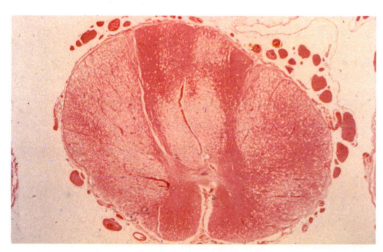

Fig. 10.7 Vacuolar myelopathy. Lower thoracic spinal cord showing marked confluent vacuolation in posterior and lateral columns, and mild-to-moderate vacuolation in anterior columns. H&E stain. Courtesy of Dr CK Petito.

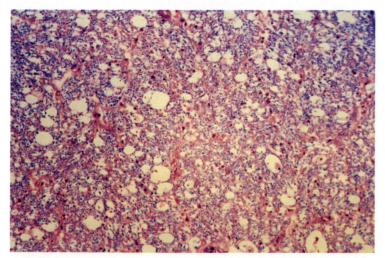

Fig. 10.8 Vacuolar myelopathy. Histological section showing demyelination and vacuolation. Luxol-fast blue stain. Courtesy of Dr MB Cohen.

Peripheral neuropathies are also common during the course of HIV infection. Acute inflammatory demyelinating polyneuropathy (Guillain–Barré syndrome – see Fig. 10.3) is usually seen at an early stage, but a more chronic form may be seen at any stage of the infection. A multiple mononeuropathy may be seen in advanced AIDS-related complex (ARC) and AIDS. The most common type of peripheral neuropathy in patients with AIDS is a distal, predominantly sensory polyneuropathy, with painful chronic symmetric dysaesthesias in a stocking distribution, most severe on the soles of the feet, sometimes accompanied by numbness and motor weakness. Electromyography shows evidence of demyelination and nerve biopsy often reveals degeneration of axons (Fig. 10.10).

Non-Hodgkin's lymphoma (NHL) involving the CNS (Figs 10.11 & 10.12) is strongly associated with AIDS. It usually presents as a single mass lesion in the brain; biopsy is necessary for definitive diagnosis. NHL in AIDS patients is usually a high-grade B-cell malignancy which exhibits aggressive biological behaviour. Histopathologically, it may be large cell, undifferentiated or immunoblastic in type (Figs 10.13 & 10.14). Epstein–Barr virus DNA sequences can be found in some but not all of these tumours.

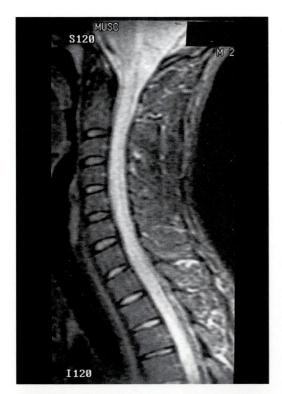 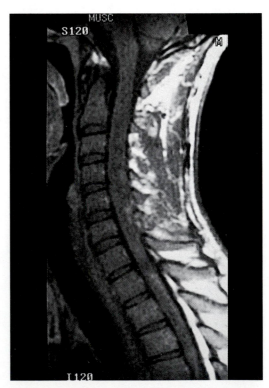

Fig. 10.9 Transverse myelitis. Left: T2-weighted sagittal MRI in an AIDS patient with transverse myelitis showing an abnormal hyperintense signal from the medulla into the upper thoracic spinal cord. Right: Post-contrast T1-weighted image demonstrating cord swelling and areas of patchy parenchymal enhancement. Courtesy of Dr P Van Tassel.

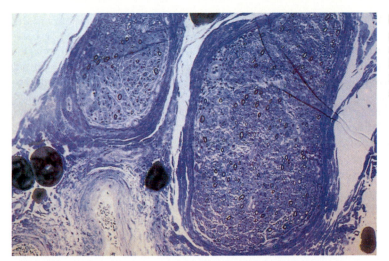

Fig. 10.10 Peripheral polyneuropathy. High power view of section of sural nerve showing severe loss of myelinated fibres and minimal inflammatory reaction. Toluidine blue stain. Courtesy of Dr HV Vinters.

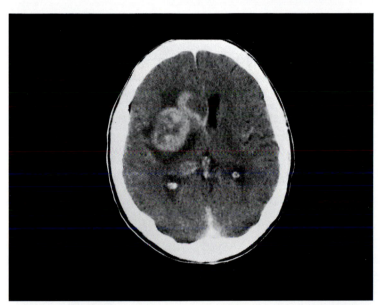

Fig.10.11 Cerebral lymphoma. CT scan showing multiple enhancing lesions of the right side of the brain due to non-Hodgkin's lymphoma in a patient with AIDS. Courtesy of Dr G Griffin.

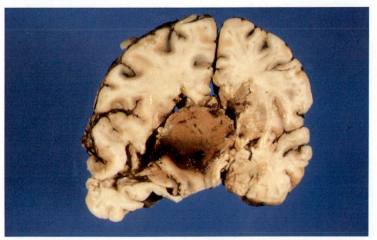

Fig. 10.12 Cerebral lymphoma. Coronal section of brain showing a firm, focally necrotic and haemorrhagic tumour mass, extending from the anterior putamen to the posterior portion of the thalamus, occupying the third ventricle and protruding laterally into the left parietal and temporal lobes. Courtesy of Dr HL Ioachim.

HUMAN T-CELL LEUKAEMIA VIRUS I

Human T-cell leukaemia virus I (HTLV-I) is a human retrovirus of the oncovirus group. Infection is most common in southern Japan and the Caribbean Basin, and among Blacks in the southeast USA. Transmission occurs from mother to child (probably via breast milk), during sexual contact (via semen), and through blood transfusion or use of contaminated needles. Infection persists for life and the virus can consistently be isolated from seropositive individuals.

The most important related human disease is adult T-cell leukaemia–lymphoma, but in endemic areas cases of a progressive neurological disease (sometimes known as tropical spastic paraplegia) have also been linked with this virus. Most of the patients have progressive bilateral spastic paraparesis, often with mild sensory involvement. Peripheral numbness or dysaesthesia, back pain and urinary frequency, urgency and incontinence are sometimes seen. Neurological examination reveals spastic paraparesis with hyperactive deep tendon reflexes. Examination of the CSF may be normal or may show slight elevation in protein concentration and mild mononuclear pleocytosis. Abnormal lymphocytes similar to those seen in adult T-cell leukaemia–lymphoma may be found in the peripheral blood or CSF, and oligoclonal protein bands, viral DNA or the complete virus may be found in the CSF. A favourable response to treatment with steroids has been seen in some patients.

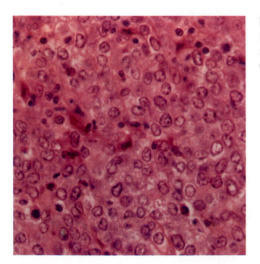

Fig. 10.13 Non-Hodgkin's lymphoma. Diffuse, undifferentiated Burkitt's cell type. Starry-sky pattern, round nuclei with fine nucleoli and numerous mitoses are seen. Haematoxylin–phloxin–saffranin stain. Courtesy of Dr HL Ioachim.

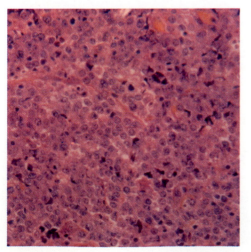

Fig. 10.14 Non-Hodgkin's lymphoma. Large, diffuse, non-cleaved cell type. Uniform large round nuclei with multiple small nucleoli and numerous mitoses are seen. Haematoxylin–phloxin–saffranin stain. Courtesy of Dr HL Ioachim.

Chapter 11

Congenital Infections

TOXOPLASMOSIS

Congenital toxoplasmosis usually results from transmission of infection to the fetus following acquisition of acute toxoplasmosis by a pregnant woman. Transmission *in utero* occasionally occurs following reactivation of chronic infection in an immunocompromised pregnant woman. If the mother develops toxoplasmosis during the first trimester the rate of transmission to the fetus is approximately 25%, and the result is usually severe disease in the newborn, spontaneous abortion or stillbirth. After the first trimester the risk of infection in the fetus is much higher, but most of the affected infants will be asymptomatic at birth. Appropriate antimicrobial treatment of the mother substantially reduces the risk of transmission of infection to the fetus. Chorioretinitis (Figs 11.1 & 11.2) is the most common manifestation of congenital toxoplasmosis, but mental and psychomotor retardation, seizure disorder, encephalitis, microcephaly, microphthalmia (Fig. 11.3), intracranial calcification (Fig. 11.4), hydrocephalus (Figs 11.5 & 11.6) and sensorineural hearing loss are also common. Most infected infants

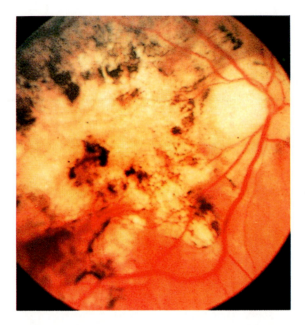

Fig. 11.1 Toxoplasmosis. Fundus photograph showing large areas of chorioretinitis with irregular scarring and pigmentation.

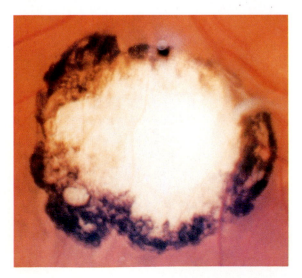

Fig. 11.2 Toxoplasmosis. Fundus photograph showing a well-defined yellow scar surrounded by pigment in healed congenital toxoplasmosis.

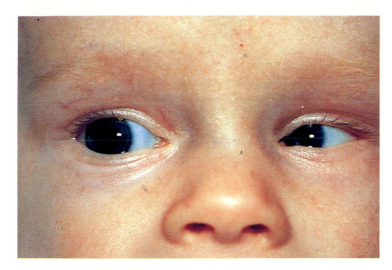

Fig. 11.3 Toxoplasmosis. Microphthalmia in congenital toxoplasmosis. Courtesy of Dr MJ Wood.

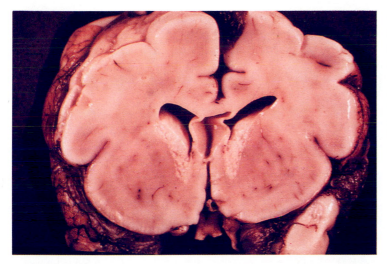

Fig. 11.4 Congenital toxoplasmosis. Brain of a premature infant revealing subependymal necrosis and calcification appearing as bilaterally symmetrical areas of whitish discolouration. The subependymal change is in the region of the caudate nucleus; the vascular congestion seen below this is probably unrelated to the primary pathological process.

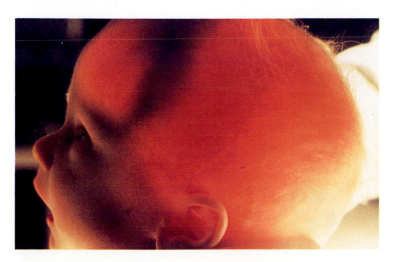

Fig. 11.5 Toxoplasmosis. Transillumination of the skull, showing severe hydrocephalus secondary to congenital toxoplasmosis. Courtesy of Dr MJ Wood.

eventually develop signs of toxoplasmosis, but these may not appear until several months after delivery. Congenital toxoplasmosis must be differentiated from rubella, cytomegalovirus infection, herpes simplex virus infection, syphilis and listeriosis. A markedly elevated protein concentration in the CSF is typical of congenital toxoplasmosis. IgG may be passively transferred from mother to fetus across the placenta, but a persistent or rising titre of IgG, or a positive test for IgM, provides evidence of infection in the infant. If toxoplasmosis is suspected in an apparently healthy newborn baby, therapy with pyrimethamine plus sulfadiazine should be administered for three weeks, followed by sulfadiazine alone until the diagnosis is confirmed or discarded. If the diagnosis is confirmed, treatment should be continued for a minimum of six months in infants who are asymptomatic at birth, and for a year if signs of infection are present.

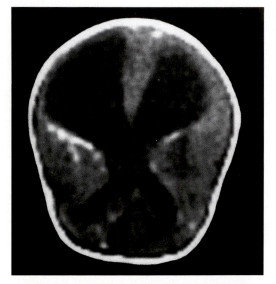

Fig. 11.6 Toxoplasmosis. CT scan of skull illustrated in Fig. 11.5, showing severe hydrocephalus and periventricular calcification. Courtesy of Dr MJ Wood.

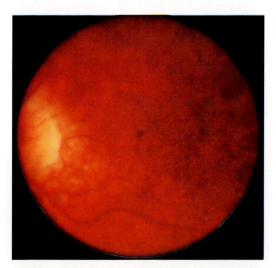

Fig. 11.7 Rubella retinopathy. Fundus photograph showing characteristic clumping of pigment and areas of retinal degeneration in the region of the macula. Courtesy of G Catford.

RUBELLA

Infants with congenital rubella shed large quantities of virus in body secretions for many months in spite of high titres of neutralizing antibody in the serum. How this persistent infection leads to the development of the specific manifestations of the congenital rubella syndrome is not completely understood. The effects of rubella virus on the fetus are closely related to the age of the fetus at the time infection occurs: the younger the fetus when infected the more severe the illness. The most common manifestations affecting the CNS and eye are meningoencephalitis, nerve deafness, cataract, chorioretinitis (Fig. 11.7), mental retardation, microcephaly and disorders of behaviour and language. Diagnosis of congenital rubella is made by demonstration of rubella virus or antigen with monoclonal antibody, or detection of a persistent or rising titre of IgG antibody, or presence of IgM antibody. Congenital rubella can be largely prevented by immunization of the population during childhood with live attenuated rubella vaccine. Although no cases of congenital rubella syndrome have been attributed to the vaccine, women are advised not to become pregnant for at least three months after receiving it.

CYTOMEGALOVIRUS

Most cases of clinically apparent cytomegalovirus infection occur in infants of primiparous mothers who had a primary infection during pregnancy. In this situation the risk of infection in the infant is approximately 50%. The risk of infection in infants born to mothers who were seropositive at the beginning of pregnancy is much lower—immunity in the mother evidently protects the baby from infection. Infection of the uterine cervix during pregnancy may result in the transmission of infection to a neonate during its passage through the birth canal. Such perinatal infections are usually asymptomatic but can be recognized when a neonate begins to secrete virus in the urine several weeks after birth. In classic fulminant congenital cytomegalovirus infection, jaundice, hepatosplenomegaly, petechial rash and evidence of multiple organ system involvement appear shortly after birth. Microcephaly, motor disability, intracerebral calcifications (Fig. 11.8), and chorioretinitis are often present. Infants who survive may exhibit nerve deafness, chronic seizure disorder and spastic quadriplegia. At present there are no established effective measures for prevention or treatment of congenital cytomegalovirus infection.

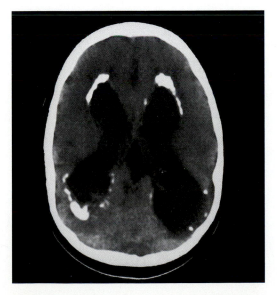

Fig. 11.8 Congenital cytomegalovirus infection. Non-contrast axial CT scan demonstrating congenital cytomegalovirus infection in the newborn. Periventricular calcifications can be seen bilaterally, along with ventriculomegaly. Courtesy of Dr P Van Tassel.